LE

STRONGER

FASTER

LOOK LIKE A FITNESS MODEL BUT PERFORM

LIKE A PROFESSIONAL ATHLETE

By

BRIAN KEANE

This book is dedicated to my mum Rita

and my daughter Holly.

CONTENTS

PROLOGUE

People always say that you should write a book you would want to read; LEANER STRONGER FASTER is exactly this. Over the course of the book, I cover everything that you would need to know as an athlete to raise your physique and performance to the next level. As someone who played Gaelic football for most of his adult life, that is the sport I reference most often throughout the book. To keep the narrative consistent, I sometimes refer to GAA (Gaelic Athletic Association) or GAA players throughout but the rules, tips and tricks apply to all athletes.

For those of you unfamiliar with Gaelic football, it is a like a mixture of rugby, soccer and basketball so a lot of the examples throughout the book apply equally well to these sports. Over the years, I have worked with everyone from GAA, soccer and rugby players to mixed martial artists and golfers and have been doing so for nearly a decade.

Although I have played sport for most of my life, I am and always have been a coach first. I have worked with thousands of amateur and professional athletes over the years so if your goal is to become leaner, stronger and faster or just to improve your energy levels, get your body fat low enough to see your abs and improve your sleep quality with some timely hacks, then this is the book for you.

How to read this book

There are two ways to approach this book. The first is the obvious, tried and tested 'start to end' manner, where you start with chapter one and read till the end. However, you can also simply skip sections as you wish to. If your nutrition is something you are currently struggling with, then you can go straight to that section and read it first. If you have no idea what supplements could help you move to the next level, then jump right into that section. I've tried to interlink the book using threads that refer back to other chapters to provide context to any given section, but I've primarily written it so that the sections stand alone and would make sense perfectly even if you're shuffling between sections. My intention for this book is for you to have it at hand to refer back to it as often as you need to. Of course, the way to the get the most from it is to read it in its entirety (it will take about three hours of total reading time from start to finish) but jump in and out as you need to. This was the book I dreamed of reading when I was still playing sport full time; so if you share a similar sense of wanting to not only play your best but also look your best, then this is the book for you. I hope you enjoy reading it as much as I enjoyed writing it.

Brian Keane
Strength and Conditioning Coach
Sports Nutritionist

CHAPTER 1:

NUTRITION FOR ATHLETES

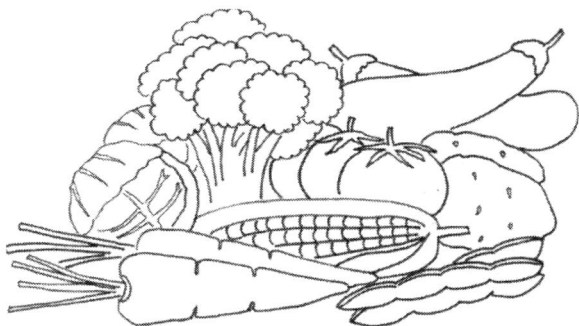

Introduction

Nutrition is your foundation for success as an athlete. Training, supplements and sleep, all have a pivotal role to play. But nothing beats getting leaner, building quality muscle or enhancing your recovery than gearing your nutrition towards your specific goals. This next section covers everything from energy, calories and macronutrients to carb cycling and the best foods for you as an athlete.

Energy for performance

When you exercise, your body needs to start producing energy much faster than it needs to at rest. The muscles start to contract more strenuously, the heart beats faster to pump blood around the body more rapidly, the lungs work harder and, as I mentioned in my first book *The Fitness Mindset*, in the case of working out at the gym, your brain begins to connect the muscles you're trying to exercise (mind-muscle connection).

I also spoke about eating the right foods to improve your energy levels in that book. The subtitle of the book – 'Eat for energy, train for tension, manage your mindset, reap the results' – is something I will expand on in greater depth in the following chapter in regard to altering your body composition as an athlete as well as improving your performance through proper fuelling and increasing your energy levels. As you probably already know, maintaining high energy levels for your gym workouts, pitch sessions and, even more importantly, your games is crucial for any athlete. So where does this energy come from? Also, how can you keep it high enough to fuel great training sessions and keep your figurative 'tank' full during big games?

What is energy?

Although we cannot actually see energy, we can feel and observe its effects in terms of heat and physical work (our output). Energy is produced by the splitting of a chemical bond in a substance called adenosine triphosphate (ATP). ATP is what allows your muscles to contract during exercise and is often referred to as the body's 'energy currency'. It is produced in every cell of the body during the breakdown of carbohydrates, fat, protein and alcohol, all of which are expanded upon in this chapter.

There are four components of food and drink that are capable of producing energy:

- Carbohydrates

- Fat

- Protein

- Alcohol

When you eat a meal or a have a drink, these components are broken down during digestion into their various building blocks, after which they are absorbed into the bloodstream. Each is expanded upon below but, to give you a brief run down, carbohydrates are broken down into small, single sugar units: glucose (the most common unit), fructose and galactose. Fats are broken down into fatty acids, while proteins are broken down into amino acids. Alcohol is mostly absorbed directly into the blood, which s one of the reasons why it's such an ineffective fuel scurce for your body.

The main purpose of all these components (the three main macronutrients and alcohol) is energy production. That being said, carbohydrates, proteins and fats also have other important functions, including supplying your body with vitamins and minerals, and they serve certain important functions as well. Regardless of the macronutrient breakdown i.e. the percentage of each macro group you are eating, such as the standard 20% fat, 20% protein and 60% carbohydrate that is generally recommended for an athlete, 'sooner or later', all food or drink components are broken down to release energy regardless of the strategy.

What is a calorie?

A calorie (or a kilocalorie) is a unit of energy. As there is some confusion regarding the difference between calories and kilocalories, I will very briefly explain this before moving on. Energy is ultimately given off by the body as heat.

- A small calorie (symbol: cal) –

1 cal is the amount of energy required to raise the temperature of one gram of water by one degree Celsius.

- A large calorie (symbol: Cal, kcal that we commonly use) –

1 Cal is the amount of energy required to raise the temperature of one kilogram of water by one degree Celsius.

1 large calorie (1kcal) = 1,000 small calories.

When we talk about calories in the everyday sense, we are actually referring to Calories, with a capital C, or kilocalories (kcal or Cal). Human beings require energy to survive – to breathe, move, pump blood, exercise, etc. – and we acquire this energy from food. The number of calories in a food item is the measure of how much potential energy that food possesses.

For example:

1 g of carbohydrates has 4 kcals of energy

1 g of protein has 4 kcals of energy

1 g of fat has 9 kcals of energy

1 g of alcohol has 7 kcals of energy

Various foods are a combination of the three main building blocks. Therefore, if you know how many carbohydrates, fats and proteins are present in any given food item, you can calculate how many calories or how much energy that food contains. Below is an example of the formula for calculating the number of calories in a food.

For example:

100 g of oats (generic brand)

This is a low-fat, high-carb, low-to-moderate-protein food.

Protein: 16.5 g (16.5 g × 4 kcal)

Carbohydrates: 66 g (66 g × 4 kcal)

Fat: 7 g (7 g × 9 kcal)

Total calories: 393 kcal

Note: The same formula can be used to calculate the number of calories in any food item. I believe that the misconception that I held throughout my early teens when first learning about macronutrients is also worth mentioning at this point. 150 g of sweet potato is not 150 g of carbohydrates; it's actually closer to 30 g of carbohydrates. The same for 50 g of oats, that's not 50 g of carbohydrate, it's actually closer to 30 g of carbohydrate. This information is important if you are calculating your own carbohydrate intake before or after matches in order to ensure optimal performance and recovery. I wanted to especially highlight it here, as it's a misconception I've had first-hand experience with and one that is shared by many athletes I have worked with.

You don't need to understand that much about calories apart from the fact that you need to be in a calorie surplus i.e. eat more calories than you burn each day to add size or gain weight, while you need to be in a calorie deficit i.e. eat less calories than you burn each day to lose fat or decrease weight. Everything else is built upon this foundation principle. In order to find your calorie maintenance (the number of calories you require to remain the same weight), you can use a simple basal metabolic rate calculator (BMR) online. These aren't 100% accurate, as they generally give you a generic recommended intake of calories based of your weight and your height while not considering your training, muscle mass or genetic make-up. However, they do give you a number to work with. If you really want a good idea of how many calories you should be eating based around your goals, it is always worth consulting a professional or sports nutritionist to determine your number. Alternatively, you can use the 'trial and error' method. For example, if you think you will lose body fat by limiting your diet to 2,000 calories a day, try eating that amount. If your body fat remains the same after a week or ten days, try reducing it to 1,900 calories and keep going till you get the desired response. As an athlete looking to get leaner or lose body fat, the goal is to lose body fat with the highest intake of calories possible. This entails that your energy levels won't be negatively affected and importantly, hunger and satiating hormones won't be downregulated due to the over-restriction of calories. It is also worth noting that you can go into a calorie deficit by virtue of your nutrition (eating less food), training (burning more calories) or a combination of the two. To add size, muscle or simply get bigger, you do the opposite. You need to eat more calories than you burn. If your goal is to get bigger and your body isn't gaining any mass, it's very likely that you're not eating enough calories. This has also been discussed at greater lengths later on in the book.

Fat is the most concentrated form of energy, providing the body with more than twice as much energy as carbohydrates or protein. However, for an athlete, it may not necessarily be the 'best' form of energy for exercise.

For example, one slice of wholegrain bread provides about the same energy (or kcals) as a large tablespoon of full-fat butter (7 g). However, their composition is very different. In bread, most of the energy (75%) comes from carbohydrates, while virtually all the energy in butter (99.7%) comes from fat.

Why a calorie isn't just a calorie!

I remember reading a quote once by Fred Stare, founder and former chair of the Harvard University Nutrition Department, that has thankfully been largely disproven since.

'Calories are all alike, whether they come from beef or bourbon (alcohol), from sugar or starch, or cheese and crackers. Too many calories are too many calories.'

To be fair, if fat loss is your primary goal, too many calories are simply too many calories regardless of whether those calories come from sugar and chocolate or chicken and turkey. However, the ways these foods are digested and absorbed are completely different. The food choices you make and the number of calories you eat will both have a huge impact on your overall body composition, performance, energy levels and health in general.

'Don't fool yourself and you're the easiest person to fool.'
– Richard Feynman

I'm usually the first to suggest that if factoring in a small amount of chocolate, sugar or even alcohol is what keeps you on track in the long term, by all means, factor that into your nutritional strategy. The only issue I have with this idea occurs when people convince themselves that a calorie is a calorie regardless of where it comes from. If you're looking to improve your energy levels, body composition and performance on the pitch, choosing higher quality foods will suit you better than a diet primarily based on beer, chocolate and pizza (as much as I wish this wasn't the case).

The truth is, it's not what you put into your mouth that matters, it's what makes it to your bloodstream. One of my mentors used to always tell me, 'It's not about what you eat, it's about what you absorb,' and the truth probably lies somewhere in the middle. Your food choices, the actual foods you put into your body, can have a massive impact on your energy levels, body composition and health in general. However, you also have to absorb the nutrients from those foods. For example, if you're intolerant to gluten or wheat, a portion of wholegrain pasta isn't going to be absorbed by your body despite it being generally considered a good carbohydrate source for most athletes. Being intolerant to a food is exactly as it sounds; your body doesn't 'tolerate' that food very well. Below, I will give you a list of high quality carbohydrate foods to experiment with, but the key is going to be testing them in your own nutritional strategy and using the sources that work best for your body i.e. testing whether they digest properly, don't sit in or bloat your stomach and give you a steady release of energy. On that note, let's get into what is arguably the most important macronutrient for any athlete – carbohydrates.

CARBOHYDRATES

The human body is designed to run on carbohydrates. While we can use protein and fat for energy, the easiest fuels for our body to use are carbohydrates. As an athlete whose training consists of sprints and lots of high-intensity work, consuming sufficient high-quality carbohydrates is crucial for maintaining as well as elevating performance and recovery.

When we eat complex carbohydrates, like whole grains, vegetables, beans and lentils, or simpler carbohydrates, like certain fruits, the body does exactly what it is designed to do – it breaks them down and produces energy. Even better, as these foods haven't been modified or processed, all the nutrients that the body requires for digestion and metabolism are already present in them. They also contain fibre, which is a less digestible type of carbohydrates that helps the digestive system run smoothly. This is one of the reasons why I am slightly biased towards whole or 'real' food as opposed to their processed alternatives. When you eat foods that come in their most natural state i.e. they haven't been altered too much, all the enzymes, vitamins and minerals required to improve their digestion and absorption are already present. This is discussed in more detail later in this chapter; but before we get to that, I would like to touch upon some of the negative associations with regard to carbohydrates.

Carbohydrates have acquired a pretty bad reputation over recent years. But when used correctly, they can be massively beneficial in keeping blood sugar levels stable, maintaining consistent energy levels and fuelling your body during tough training sessions and games. The kinds of carbohydrate choices you will make pretty much come down to your metabolism and personal digestion; for example, as mentioned before, if you don't tolerate gluten very well, wholegrain bread will be a terrible food choice for you and will actually cause more problems than it resolves (low energy, sleep interruption, increased inflammation that can lead to injury – just to name a few). On the other hand, if you tolerate it just fine, a wholegrain sandwich with some chicken or turkey at lunchtime may fit tremendously well into your lifestyle and schedule. In this section, I will guide you through different food combinations and choices but, as I mentioned earlier, the key is to experiment with different food options, figure out what works for you and then add those to your personal nutritional strategy.

Remember, carbohydrates have only one job – to give you energy. There is no 'essential carbohydrate'. There are 'essential amino acids' in protein or 'essential fatty acids' in fat, where essential entails that you need to get them from food or supplements because your body can't function properly without them. Carbohydrates exist to supply your body and brain with energy. In the case of an athlete, they also fuel your workouts and help you refuel after training as well as games, leading to improved recovery.

Why do we need carbohydrates?

- Body's main source of fuel – glucose and glycogen (stored carbs).

- Easily used by the body for energy – fuelling intensive pitch sessions and games.

- Used by all tissues and cells for energy – glucose.

- Can be stored in the muscles and liver – used later for energy.

Note: This is great for athletes and is discussed more in the 'carb loading' section

- Good source of fibre – certain types of carbohydrates that our body can't digest are passed through the intestinal tract intact and help to move waste out of the body.

How does my body store carbohydrates?

Carbohydrates are stored as glycogen in the muscles and liver, along with about three times their own weight in water; this is one of the reasons that fighters, boxers and bodybuilders reduce their carbohydrate intake before competitions if they need to make a weight class. This is also the main reason that people who switch from high-carb to low-carb diets lose a lot of weight within the first few days. They normally deplete glycogen and lose water weight instead of just body fat in most cases.

If you have ever gone 'low carb' for a few days and felt 'leaner' or have found all your clothes have become looser – this is probably why. I remember when I was in college; if I wanted to look leaner for a night out or event, I used to cut all my carbohydrates for two or three days – I would normally start on a Tuesday for a Thursday student night (author note: I do not recommend this!). However, lo and behold, my jeans would be loose, my skin felt tighter and I thought I looked great. Then, Friday night's training session would come and my energy would be zapped; any niggle or strain felt ten times worse, and as soon as I went back to eating normally, I would go back to looking exactly as I had on Tuesday. At the time, I didn't understand the connection between carbohydrates, performance and weight or fat loss.

In reality, going low carb for a few days can really support you if fat loss is one of your primary goals. I actually keep some of the athletes that I train on low-carbohydrate diets during their rest days. We then cycle up or increase it to a moderate intake of carbohydrates on normal training days and load on the day before and on the day of games or particularly intense training sessions. So, low carbohydrates definitely can have an application for certain players but, at the time, I just didn't understand how to use low-carb diets, which led to my performance being affected. To be honest, I didn't really understand the difference between body fat and weight for years; I thought they were the same thing.

Losing 'weight' and losing 'body fat' is not the same thing. To lose weight is to reduce numbers on a scale i.e. you weigh 80 kg and lose 3 kg. While your new weight is 77 kg, your body fat and your body composition may look exactly the same as they did at 80 kg. But since the numbers on the scale have dropped, it's considered 'losing weight'. Reducing body fat, on the other hand, is as it sounds. It's reducing the amount of fat in your body – you can drop two full jeans sizes and look significantly leaner without losing any weight! At times, you will definitely get both – you will lose body fat and weight together – but it's not always the case. If you're looking to lose body fat, your goal should be reducing the fat on your body and not lowering a number on a scale. If fat loss s one of your primary goals, one of my intentions with this book is to help you reduce body fat while keeping your fuel tanks full, taking your performance to the next level. If muscle building or getting bigger is one of your primary goals, I will also be covering that later in the book.

Glycogen explained

There is about three times more glycogen stored in the muscles than in the liver. Glycogen is a large molecule, similar to starch, and is made up of many glucose units joined together. However, the body can only store a relatively small amount of glycogen; it doesn't have a limitless supply. Storing and loading your glycogen before big games and training sessions is crucial for performance. Think about it this way – stored glycogen is like petrol or diesel for your car; it's your body's main fuel source. You wouldn't drive from Cork to Dublin,

Birmingham to London or New York to Chicago without filling up your gas tank before leaving. Glycogen stores before a game function much in the same way.

The total store of glycogen in the average body amounts to about 500 g, with approximately 400 g in the muscles and 100 g in the liver. Again, this can vary depending on your bodyweight and your metabolism, but it's a pretty reliable number to start with. On carb-loading days, you may need to increase or decrease your intake depending on your body type; for example, if you have an extremely fast metabolism, you may have to double your intake of carbohydrate to 1,000g to have an effective pre-game carb load. For the average player, this store is equivalent to 1,600-2,000 kcals or so, which means that it's worth consuming this volume of calories from carbohydrates on the day before games to seriously top up your fuel stores.

Do carbs make me fat?

Like most things in life, there isn't a simple 'yes' or 'no' answer to this question. Fat is stored as adipose (fat) tissue in almost every region of the body. Sometimes, it feels like you hold it more in certain places than others, and while this may be true, there will be some amount of fat in most places on your body in general. It may simply be more pronounced around your stomach, lower back or hips (discussed below). This can sometimes be either genetic, based cn your food choices or, in some instances, even come down to the natural testosterone level in your body if you're male. This is expanded upon in the testosterone section of the book.

While there's a small amount of fat stored in the muscles, the majority is stored around the organs and beneath the skin. Unfortunately, there is little you can do to change how your body distributes fat. So, if your stomach or lower back is your 'stubborn area', i.e. the last bit of body fat that gets processed for energy, you can't really change this. However, you can definitely alter the *amount* of fat that is stored, which is much more important and completely in your control. You can't control to which areas your body distributes its fat, but you have full control over how much fat you have in your body. This starts with unde-standing the power of carbohydrates and how best to utilise them in your nutritional strategy.

The power of carbs for athletes

Carbohydrate is required to fuel almost every type of activity, and the amount of glycogen stored in the muscles and liver has a direct effect on your performance at the gym, on the pitch and during a game. Keeping your glycogen stores full can enable you to train at your optimal intensity in the gym and on the pitch. The analogy I return to is that of the fuel in a car – if your car runs out of fuel, it will cease to function almost instantly. Keeping your glycogen stores topped up for games is very similar – it's your fuel. If your muscle glycogen is too low, it will lead to early fatigue, reduced training intensity and significantly lower cognitive performance (reaction times) in some cases. Here are some of the common mistakes that athletes make when it comes to carbohydrates. I know this because I have made them all as well.

Mistake #1: Eating like a bodybuilder

This was probably where I committed the biggest mistake; I didn't realise that eating for performance was very different from eating for aesthetics or 'to look good'. When I started bodybuilding at seventeen, i.e. building my body, I also followed the bodybuilding diets that were popular at the time, which were generally low-carb, moderate-fat and high-protein diets. I was pretty much an 'if the magazine says it's true, then it must be true' kind of guy and followed each diet gram for gram.

Granted, it did work. I got significantly leaner and a bit bigger, but my performance on the pitch suffered dramatically; I went from playing county underage, making top college teams and being a regular starter for my senior club to struggling to make every single team, all in the space of about eighteen months. Why? What had happened? Well for one, my training was completely out of sync with my goals, which lead to a whole range of injuries, but more importantly, my energy levels had dramatically dropped from the lack of carbohydrates in my diet and impacted my performance and concentration on the pitch. Although I didn't know it at the time, the answer was pretty straightforward. I wanted to be leaner, a bit bigger, have a six pack and improve my performance on the pitch, but my nutrition (particularly my carbohydrate intake) was not in alignment with the goals I was looking to accomplish.

Clearly then, glycogen is the most important and most valuable fuel for any type of exercise? Well, yes and no. Following exercise, glycogen stores will require replenishing as a key part of your recovery process. The easiest and most straightforward way of achieving this is by consuming a high-carbohydrate diet. For most athletes, that's an intake of 5-10 g of carbs for each kilo of bodyweight i.e. 400-800g of carbs for an athlete who weighs 80 kg. However, this is just a general rule and doesn't necessarily consider body composition or how you actually look. It also doesn't account for insulin sensitivity or how efficiently your body converts carbohydrates into energy either. If you don't care about how you look, then this is a decent number to start from. Although, if you're looking to alter your body composition **and** improve performance, try this instead.

What to Do:

Honestly, it's only in the last eight or nine years of working on myself and with the thousands of athletes that I've coached over the years, from professional fitness models and bodybuilders to club and elite county players, that I've learnt the difference between how to eat for performance and how to eat 'to look good'. Even though your body can convert protein to glucose (a process called gluconeogenesis), it's a terrible energy source for a sprint sport athlete; it's like putting really cheap gas in your car. It will surely move, but it's likely to break down five miles into the journey. Protein is not usually a major source of energy, but it can be used as a fuel source when glycogen stores are exhausted. During a period of consistent low-carb diets, glycogen would be in short supply. This would cause more proteins to be broken down into glucose in order to provide the body with fuel. Even when I first heard about this at the age of seventeen, I thought that if I depleted my glycogen stores by following a low-carb diet, it would force my body to break down fat and use that as a fuel source. Unfortunately, this isn't always the case If you don't refuel your glycogen stores regularly, not only are you using an inadequate fuel source for your body but you also risk losing muscle. This has negative consequences regardless of your goal. If building muscle or getting bigger is your primary goal, the negatives are obvious – you will have less muscle and become smaller. However, if fat loss is your primary goal, losing or burning through lean muscle tissue can be just as problematic. The more lean muscle tissue you have, the potentially higher your metabolism will be i.e. you will burn more calories throughout the day. A loss of lean muscle tissue can thereby reduce the number of calories you burn throughout the day. The good news is that this is pretty easily avoidable, and there is a simple, straightforward nutritional system that you can apply right away. It's called carb cycling.

Carb Cycling

Carb cycling is effectively when you cycle (reduce or increase) your carbohydrates intake on different days. A simple break down of this is presented as follows:

- Low on rest days (assuming you don't have a game the following day)

- Moderate on training days (gym or pitch training)

- High on the day before and day of games or big training sessions (game day or your weekly leg workout in the off season)

The numbers vary greatly from person to person and greatly depend on your training program, your metabolism and your training schedule in general. Just to give you a range, I've had some of my players go with 50 g of carbs on low days, 150 g on moderate and 300 g on high days, while others have used 200 g on low days, 400 g on moderate days and 800 g on high days. To keep it simple to follow, I'm going to use 100 g for low days, 200 g for moderate and 300 g for high days as the volumes going forward.

Carb cycling with complex carbs

Carbohydrates are traditionally classified according to their chemical structure. The most simplistic method classifies them into two categories: simple (sugars) and complex (starches and fibres). These terms simply refer to the number of sugar units in the molecule. Simple carbohydrates are extremely small molecules consisting of one or two sugar units. They comprise of monosaccharaides (one sugar unit, 'mono' means one), namely glucose (dextrose, which is present in many sports performance drinks), fructose (fruit sugar) and galactose (found in milk), and disaccharides (two sugar units, 'di' means two), which include sucrose (normal table sugar, which is a mixture of glucose and fructose) and lactose (milk sugar that is a mixture of glucose and galactose). Lactose intolerance is the inability to break down sugar lactose. If you are lactose intolerant, you can potentially supplement it with lactase (the enzyme needed to break down lactose). However, I would consider avoiding it completely.

Note: This doesn't mean you can't supplement with whey protein; it just means you need to choose a whey protein that doesn't contain any lactose.

Complex carbohydrates are much larger molecules that consist of ten to several thousand sugar units (mostly glucose) joined together. They include the starches amylose and amylopectin as well as the non-starch polysaccharides (dietary fibres), such as cellulose, pectin and hemicellulose.

In between simple and complex carbohydrates are glucose polymers and maltodextrin, which comprise of 3-10 sugar units. They are produced due to the partial breakdown of corn starch during food processing. They are traditionally used as bulking and thickening agents in processed foods such as sauces, desserts, soda drinks, etc. and have become very popular in the sports drink community owing to their low sweetness level and high energy density compared to sucrose or regular table sugar. Personally, I'm not a massive fan of maltodextrin as I believe there are more effective alternatives. However, if it's factored in as part of a good nutritional strategy, it can effectively serve as a supplement as long as you don't use it as a 'quick fix' carb supplement for supplying you with energy. If your energy levels are consistently low, it's normally indicative of something being off in your nutrition, recovery or sleep pattern, and using a supplement simply acts as a 'plaster' for the problem. My personal philosophy, which provides my athletes with longevity, is to get your nutrition, sleep and recovery on point and then use your supplements to move from a figurate performance level of a nine to a ten instead of going from a two to a four.

Personally, I rarely use maltodextrin before, during or after workouts for the majority of my players – particularly for those who are sensitive, with food intolerances or allergies, but it can definitely serve a purpose. If you decide to incorporate it into your nutritional plan, I would suggest starting with a small dose (10-20 g) and gradually building up to see how your body responds to it. If you find it's helping you on game days or during your more intense training sessions, then continue consuming it. If it's causing you stomach discomfort or isn't improving performance, stick with good complex carbohydrates from food and maybe some simple sugars right before training sessions or games instead.

In practice, many foods contain a mixture of both simple and complex carbohydrates, making the traditional classification of food as 'simple' and 'complex' extremely confusing. Similar to the oats example from the calorie section, the nutritional 'majority rules' tend to apply here as well; for example, if a food is mostly made up of complex carbs (oats, sweet potato, brown rice), we call it a complex carb, while if it's mostly made up of simple sugars (cakes, biscuits, etc.), we normally call it a simple sugar.

There's a time and place for different types of carbohydrates and the Pareto Principle 80:20 rule works extremely well here. I try and get my athletes to obtain 80% of their intake from complex carbohydrates (breakfast, before, during and after training as well as most meals during carb load days) and 20% from simple sugars (right before a game, half time or as a 'free/cheat' meal during the week). This varies from player to player but tends to work well for most athletes.

Although it's tempting to think that simple carbohydrates, due to their smaller molecular size, are absorbed more quickly than complex carbohydrates and produce a rapid rise in blood sugar, this isn't always the case. For example, many starchy foods (complex carbohydrates), such as white potatoes and white bread, are digested and absorbed extremely quickly and cause a rapid rise in blood sugar. With the exception of right before, during or after games, spiking your blood sugar is generally best avoided.

Another misleading food (that contains simple carbohydrates) is apples; although a fruit, apples produce a small and prolonged rise in blood sugar despite being high in simple carbohydrates. They contain a certain type of fibre called pectin, which is

32

found between the cell walls of plants and is classified as soluble fibre. Soluble fibres have been seen to slow down digestion by attracting water and forming a gel that ultimately helps you feel fuller for longer and provides you with a steadier release of energy. This makes it a great 'on the go' snack during the day.

Simple sugars definitely have a time and place in certain programs. If you find that a quick simple sugar energy hit before a game or at half-time helps your performance, factoring this in could support you massively, provided that you have already topped up your glycogen stores with complex carbohydrates.

To confuse things further, while most fruits spike blood sugars, not all do so. Similarly, most potatoes and breads spike blood sugars but sweet potatoes or wholegrain bread do not. What's more important, as far as sports performance is concerned, is how rapidly the carbohydrates are absorbed from the small intestine into your blood stream. The faster these transfer, the more rapidly the carbohydrates can be used by the muscle cells and make a difference to your training, performance and recovery. The system that effectively allowed me to wrap my head around this was that of the glycaemic index.

The glycaemic index

To describe the effect different foods have on your blood sugar levels more accurately, scientists developed the glycaemic index (GI). The differences between carbohydrate foods can be described in terms of their GI. Simply put, this index, which ranges from 0 to 100, indicates how quickly a food raises blood sugar levels. Glucose is rated at 100, and the closer to 100 a food is rated, the more it affects blood sugar levels.

Anita Bean, in her book *The Complete Guide to Sports Nutrition*, explains this concept using an example of a baked potato. For example, to test baked potatoes, you would eat 250 g of potatoes, which contain 50 g of carbohydrates. Over the next two hours, a sample of blood is taken every fifteen minutes and the blood sugar is measured. The blood sugar is plotted on a graph and the area under the curve is calculated. Your response to the test food (e.g. potato) is compared with your blood sugar response to 50 g of glucose (the reference food). The GI is given as a percentage, which is calculated by dividing the area under the curve after you've eaten potatoes by the area under the curve after you've eaten the glucose. Thus, if the GI of baked potatoes is 85, it means that consuming a baked potato produces a rise in blood sugar that is 85% of that produced by consuming an equivalent amount of glucose.

The GI of more than 600 foods is known and, although you definitely don't need to know all 600, it helps to know about a few of the low GI, slow-digesting complex carbs in order to allow you to factor your favourite ones into your plan. I've found that my athletes tend to find it easier to classify foods as having a high GI (60-100), medium GI (40-59) and low GI (less than 40).

- <u>Low-GI complex carbohydrates</u>: oats, quinoa, brown rice, wholegrain bread, wholegrain pasta (the day before and day of games)

- <u>High-GI simple sugars</u>: dextrose, glucose (before, during or after training)

- <u>Medium GI:</u> maltodextrin, if you can tolerate it (before, during or after training), apples, pineapple, baked potatoes

- Avoid (if possible): white bread, white pasta, white rice

This isn't to say that there aren't more or better options; these are just some of my personal favourites and are easily available in most places.

It's worth noting that the speed at which blood sugar levels can rise also depends on the food combinations in a meal. For example, having a simple sugar with a fat source will slow down the speed at which it raises blood sugar. So, it's worth knowing this if you plan to have some glucose or dextrose before, during or after training. It's best to consume it by itself or with a fast-absorbing form of protein (whey protein for example) so that its speed of absorption isn't negatively affected. This won't matter too much if you are eating low-GI and slowly digesting carbs, as eating a fat or protein source with it may slow down its absorption further and won't have any negative effect on your digestion or carb load.

Slow-digesting carbs before training

Whether to eat high-GI or low-GI food before training has long been a controversial subject. Some scientific studies and anecdotal evidence swear by having simple sugars before training, while others swear by eating complex carbs before training. Again, the truth is probably somewhere in the middle. Some people work better with fast carbohydrates before training, some perform better with slow carbohydrates before training, and some with a combination of both. Although, I recommend experimenting and figuring out what works best for you. The majority of athletes who I work with find the combination works great for them. They have high-quality complex carbohydrates on the day before a game as well as on the day of the game, have simple sugars right before a game and at half time and then have complex carbs as their post-workout or post-game meal.

As I suggested before, experiment with your own strategy, timings and intake to see what works best for you. The advice I will offer you though, never experiment with new foods or nutritional strategies for the first time before or during games. I will never forget this college game where we were playing UCD (University College Dublin) in Sligo. The corner-forward who played inside me had tried some new carb energy drink from a local health store before the game and about twenty minutes into the first half, he was begging the coaches to take him off because he needed to use the toilet. They wouldn't take him off and kept telling him it was nearly half-time. Then, about five minutes before half-time, he ran the length of the pitch, past every single player, past the referee and fans in the stand and headed straight for the toilet in the dressing room. It was the fastest I've ever seen him (or anyone for that matter) run during a game! Needless to say, he never used that carb drink again. The lesson here is always experiment with different foods, nutritional strategies and supplements during training sessions and not games. Experiment with one small change at a time – a small amount of a new food or supplement and see how your body reacts to it. When you find what works best for you, then you can apply it to your game-day strategy.

PROTEIN

Proteins are made of varying combinations of amino acids. There are twenty in total – eight essential, meaning we need to get them from food or supplements, and twelve non-essential, meaning our bodies can make them from the other amino acids we consume.

Amino acids make up every tissue and substance in our bodies, from our hair and heart to our hormones. Depending on your goals, in order to build a leaner or more muscular body and improve recovery on the pitch, we require the right combination of amino acids interacting with fundamentally healthy cells in order to repair and build tissues for lean muscle.

Carbohydrates and fats are important, but nothing compares to the ability of amino acids to grow, repair and maintain healthy tissues.

The eight essential amino acids:

1.   Valine

2.   Isoleucine

3.   Leucine

4. Phenylalanine

5. Threonine

6. Tryptophan

7. Methionine

8. Lysine

The twelve non-essential amino acids:

1. Alanine

2. Arginine

3. Asparagine

4. Aspartic Acid

5. Cysteine

6. Glutamic Acid

7. Glutamine

8. Glycine

9. Histidine (essential for babies, not adults)

10. Proline

11. Serine

12. Tyrosine

Animal and fish protein contains all the essential amino acids in proper proportions to each other – a characteristic shared by all flesh foods – and is thus known as the complete protein. You can also acquire essential amino acids in the plant kingdom; they are just not in their complete protein proportions and therefore, you have to mix and match them to effectively have complete proteins. Because most plants provide inadequate amounts of certain amino acids in relation to others, plant protein is normally referred to as 'incomplete' protein.

For what do we need protein?

• Growth – especially when looking to build lean muscle tissue

• Tissue repair – to repair muscle tissue after intensive workouts and games

• Immune function – to avoid falling ill

• To obtain energy when carbohydrates are not available – this is done through gluconeogenesis, whereby your body converts protein to glucose for energy. As mentioned earlier, this is not a great fuel source for an athlete and is best avoided by carb loading before a game (explained above in the carbohydrate section).

- To preserve lean muscle mass – to retain the muscle you already have

Your protein choice

Your muscles consume and spend more protein than any other tissue. They demand a quantity of protein that is at least equivalent to that lost/utilised in a day. If your daily protein intake is insufficient, your muscles may not be getting the amino acids that they require to grow or repair themselves. However, not eating enough protein (or calories in general) isn't the only way that your muscles break down. The protein food choices you make are just as important. The choices you make should include complete protein sources that include all the essential amino acids and should be from quality sources so their absorption can be maximised.

What to look for in protein foods

Your muscle requires a protein food that is complete and wholesome. It should contain all the key amino acids along with nutritional cofactors such as naturally occurring vitamins, minerals, and antioxidants. Ideally, the food you choose to fulfil your protein requirement should be fresh, minimally processed, chemical-free and easily digestible. In its whole food form, protein is always attached to its naturally occurring cofactors, such as minerals, vitamins and carbs or fats in some cases. I would suggest that you try and avoid pre-packaged meats as much as possible. Sometimes, especially 'on the go', they can be better than nothing, but they shouldn't be a staple in your nutrition.

Meat and fish as complete proteins

Technically, all animal flesh and marine foods, including meat, poultry, eggs, dairy, fish and seafood, are complete proteins and should all suit your muscle and recovery requirements. Plant foods, on the other hand, are considered incomplete and inferior choices, as they don't contain all the essential amino acids that your body requires.

How do I get my protein if I don't eat meat?

It's true that meat and eggs are complete proteins, especially in contrast to beans and nuts. However, we don't require every essential amino acid from every meal we eat – we only need a sufficient amount of each amino acid each day. During the digestive process, our bodies liberate the amino acids present in our food and produce other substances from them. According to the Centres for Disease Control and Prevention, if something we eat doesn't contain all the essential amino acids required by the body, we have a small window (about a day) to ingest the complementary ones that complete the amino-acid equation.

The body doesn't house or store amino acids (i.e. you need to eat them every day), but as long as you eat the correct food combinations during the day, you will be fine. As mentioned above, you don't necessarily have to combine them in one meal. You just need to ensure that you combine the right foods to get all the essential amino acids in the correct amounts by the end of the day. There are numerous ways to use food combinations to obtain all your essential amino acids. I'll list a few examples below.

Combining nuts and seeds with legumes or grains

Combining legumes with sunflower seeds, sesame seeds or nuts, such as walnuts, almonds or cashews, provides complete proteins. One of my personal favourites is a trail mix of nuts, cashews and sunflower seeds with hummus or guacamole dip and raw vegetables.

To cement the idea that you do not need to consume protein-rich food together in a single meal in order to reap the benefits of combining proteins, the University of Michigan's reports state that, 'Eating a variety of foods with incomplete proteins throughout the day allows your body to get the amino acids you need from diet.' The one thing to remember is that your body doesn't store complete proteins for a rainy day. According to the Standing Committee on the Scientific Evaluation for Dietary Reference Intakes, 'There is no evidence for a protein reserve that serves only as a store to meet future needs', which means you need to stay on top of your nutrition and combine your foods every single day to reap all the benefits of essential amino acids. However, once you use the correct nutritional strategy, which includes all the essential amino acids, you can acquire all the benefits of a complete protein eater, as long as you are resourceful with your combinations.

If you're vegan, your best options are the proper

combinations of plant foods such as legumes and seeds (hummus), legumes and nuts, peas and potatoes, and beans and grains. Note that sprouted beans and grains yield a higher nutritional value and faster nutrient delivery than their conventional equivalents. However, legumes, seeds, nuts and grains are digested and assimilated slowly. Additionally, even though these foods are whole and healthy, they aren't as efficient as whey protein for muscle nourishment during the day, and they're certainly not as effective in promoting muscle recovery after training. If you are vegan, I strongly suggest you consider adding a high quality rice or hemp protein to your pre and post-workout nutrition. Try and use one that that has all the essential amino acids and consider adding an additional 5-10 g of BCAAs to it in the form of powder, capsules or tablets. Vegan proteins have decent nutritional profiles, but BCAAs (which are crucial for post-workout recovery, see below) aren't their strong suit.

Whey protein post workout

Animal flesh and marine foods are slow to digest and slow to assimilate or absorb, which makes them suboptimal for muscle recovery after training or games.

After exercise, your muscles require fast assimilating proteins. Only fast assimilating or absorbing proteins can swiftly block the catabolic effect of exercise and shift your muscle into an anabolic state. Slow-digesting proteins such as meat and fish, although great at other times of the day, don't fulfil your muscle requirements as efficiently after training.

Whey protein is a by-product of cheese manufacturing. It was initially discarded as waste or used for animal feed, but later scientists discovered that it was an outstandingly beneficial food. The nutritional properties of whey are truly remarkable. But to make use of them, you have to be careful about the whey protein that you choose. Not all whey products are the same.

Unfortunately, a lot of whey products today are derived from ultra-pasteurised milk and are loaded with preservatives, additives and sweeteners that render absorption less effective. This basically means that low-quality whey protein can make you feel sick after drinking it.

I remember the first time I drank whey protein was when I was seventeen. It was a cheap tub from some health store and it was the only one I could afford at the time. The first time I had it, within thirty minutes of drinking it, I remember my stomach looking like I was six months pregnant! Safe to say that I couldn't finish the tub and, as cheap as it was, it ended up being more expensive because I gave it away for free. My take-home message is to either buy good quality whey protein or stick to whole foods. As good as whey protein is, it's still just a supplement. It will 'supplement' what you're missing from your nutrition and, despite having great recovery benefits, is by no means essential.

Other side effects of poor whey proteins include bloating and acne on your skin from increased inflammation or a negative response to some of the added sweeteners or preservatives. If you are experiencing any of these side effects, you may not be digesting the amino acids from that supplement and should consider discontinuing its use. Not only are you wasting your money and bloating your stomach but you could also be potentially experiencing a negative effect from the absorption of other micro and macronutrients that you're consuming around the same time. Consistent bloating is a direct feedback to your body that you're not able to tolerate the food or supplement properly. If possible, try and minimise all supplements and foods that cause such effects.

I'm not going to recommend any particular brand as there are some very reputable companies out there, alongside some that are not so reputable, so be sure to do your own due diligence when buying whey protein.

However, when choosing your whey protein, the three rules that I follow are listed below:

1.   Choose one that you digest well i.e. doesn't make you feel ill or bloated after drinking it.

2.   Choose one you enjoy the taste of. There are so many great tasting whey proteins on the market that there's no reason for you to not enjoy the taste of the one you choose.

3.   Choose one that fits into your budget. The most expensive one isn't necessarily the best quality, but price is usually a good indicator of value in this case. If you can buy a cheap tub for half the price of a well-known brand, it might be a sign that it uses significantly poorer ingredients.

Money-saving tip

My top tip is to try some samples of whey proteins before you buy a tub. Most companies and supplement stores have sample sachets from different brands and are happy to give them to anyone who asks. Try a few different ones, see which one you like the best and then buy a full tub of it. This way, you won't make the same mistake I did by buying the biggest tub I could afford, using it three or four times and ther giving the rest away for free.

Why is whey protein so good?

Personally, I'm a big fan of other protein sources, such as rice and hemp protein, especially to mix up my amino acid profile intake during the year. However, pound for pound, the protein profile in whey is more impressive than any other food on the planet. It provides the largest spectrum of essential and non-essential amino acids, and it contains a remarkably high amount of the muscle building and recovery enhancing branched-chain amino acids (BCAAs). In particular, it contains leucine, which is the powerhouse of all the amino acids in terms of muscle building and recovery.

One of whey protein's most important properties is fast nutrient delivery. This trait makes whey protein most suitable for muscle recovery after exercise. As mentioned above, after exercise, your muscles are at their peak capacity of utilising nutrients, and this is when you need to feed them with fast assimilating nutrients. This is true for post-match nutrition as well as post-gym training. Whey protein can perfectly accommodate this window of opportunity. It can yield the fastest anabolic impact for your muscles.

Post-exercise recovery meals

Personally, I've been a victim of focusing too much on my 'pre-game' meals in the past and always asking myself questions like, 'What's the most important thing to eat before a game?' or, 'What should I be eating the day before a game?' and while these are great questions to ponder over, they do not address/include the full picture. The importance of recovery meals is often overlooked or misunderstood; yet, knowing how and when to incorporate a recovery meal into your strategy can make a massive difference in your overall recovery, strength or muscle gains. The main functions of post-exercise recovery, after training, games and the gym are listed as follows:

-    Promote actual growth by stimulating natural growth and steroidal hormones

-    Prevent muscle breakdown and enhance recovery

There are some myths in the gym world regarding the 'anabolic window'. It's considered the period after you train during which your body requires amino acids and carbohydrates. If the body doesn't get these, 'the workout is considered wasted'. Depending on the

51

studies you read or the people you talk to, you will hear claims supporting and negating both sides and again, the truth probably lies somewhere in between.

The one thing that is certain is that your body and muscles are like a 'sponge', soaking up macronutrients, vitamins and minerals after your train. So, taking advantage of this post-exercise window of opportunity can seriously enhance your recovery and has the potential to change your body composition even faster – considering everything else in your nutritional plan, of course.

There is a period of about thirty minutes after you train when all the lactic acid has cleared and your body's growth and recovery promoting hormone reaches its peak levels, while insulin reaches its peak sensitivity. This is precisely when meals should be ingested. At this time, muscle possesses its highest potential to assimilate nutrients, recuperate and grow (by increasing protein utilisation in the muscle).

'Right nutrition at the right time equals maximum recuperation and facilitation of muscular development.'

– Ori Holfmeklear

In other words, what you eat and when you eat is everything when it comes to optimising your post-workout nutrition.

To actually promote an immediate recuperating effect, you should take full advantage of this window of opportunity and, theoretically, ingest your recovery meal during the first thirty minutes after intense exercise. My favourite choice for such meals is a high-quality protein supplement that floods your muscles with the amino acids it requires immediately after training.

Nevertheless, after prolonged intense drills, I recommend waiting thirty to sixty minutes before ingesting a recovery shake or meal. The reason for this being that prolonged intense drills (such as metabolic conditioning style gym workouts) cause an accumulation of lactic acid in the muscles as well as the liver, which can potentially lead to a temporary state of insulin resistance, not allowing your body to absorb the nutrients as efficiently. Personally, I've made this mistake on several occasions – trying to consume a shake or meal directly after intense metabolic conditioning workouts. Let's just say, the meal didn't even reach my digestive system, let alone get absorbed.

This waiting period lets the body clear the lactic acid and regain insulin sensitivity. Thereafter, it is optimal to have your recovery meal. I would recommend you base your post-workout meal or shake timing on your training program. If you are following a recovery strategy, such as stretching at the end of a pitch session, gym workouts or games, you're effectively clearing that lactic acid during that time; thus, you can have your post-workout shake or meal as soon as you reach the dressing room. However, if you have just finished a round of 100m sprints or a metabolic conditioning workout, I would suggest waiting the thirty minutes or so.

Personally, by analysing my own recovery and by tracking and monitoring hundreds of my clients over the past few years, I've found that a post-workout recovery meal should be a blend of fast-releasing proteins first, followed by a complex carbohydrate with a slow-releasing protein source. The fast-releasing protein, such as whey protein, will help boost an immediate post-exercise protein synthesis, whereas the slow release protein in the follow-up meal will help sustain the already established anabolic or recovery state in the muscle tissue.

Some athletes find that a fast-releasing carbohydrate source after training (such as glucose or dextrose) works tremendously well for speeding up their recovery. The fast-releasing carbohydrates can be optimal for inducing an insulin spike and kick-starting the replenishing of glycogen stores. Personally, I'm not a fan of spiking blood sugars post workout, but it definitely has its importance for some athletes and is worth experimenting with to gauge what works best for you and your body. If you find having some simple sugars after you train improves your recovery and you feel great two hours later, then continue to include them in your recovery meal. On the other hand, if you feel a little sick thirty minutes later or your energy levels crash two hours afterwards, then maybe stick to having only whey protein directly after training and complex carbohydrates as well as a slow-digesting protein source in your post-workout meal. Additionally, if fat loss is your primary goal, I would consider limiting simple sugars altogether.

Directly after training: 30-50 g of whey protein (potentially add 30-50 g of dextrose)

Thirty minutes after training: 250 g of sweet potatoes and 150 g of chicken

There are loads of other food combinations that you can use, and you can substitute any complex carb and easily digestible complete protein source. Post-exercise recovery meals should be practical, handy and readily available after a workout, so carry your shake (and even your meal if required) with you to training, the gym and matches. As important as your pre-workout and pre-game meals are, your post-workout nutrition is equally as important.

Side note about refuelling and muscle damage:

Muscle damage, either through direct body contact and bruising from games or eccentric loading in the gym (activities that make you sore a day later or give you DOMS – delayed onset muscle soreness), causes a delay in the replenishment of glycogen stores. Running and sprinting in games involves eccentric muscle contraction and a single hard or intense game or training session may cause significant disruptions of muscle fibres, which physically interferes with their glycogen storing capacity. Furthermore, the white blood cells (that protect your body from getting sick) that rush to the area as part of the immune system's 'mopping up' brigade use glucose, glycogen's precursors, as their own fuel. This is why it's so important to properly refuel after intense training and gym sessions or after playing a game, so your immune system doesn't become comprised and lead you to feel run down or sick. Some studies have shown that problems with glycogen stores following muscle damage can be at least partially overcome by increasing carbohydrate intake during the 24-hour post-session window. Therefore, if you have completed a particular gruelling training session or game where a lot of muscle damage has occurred, it's worth paying extra attention to your nutrition strategy during the first 24 hours and eating additional high-carbohydrate foods may help speed up your recovery, preventing you from falling sick. I have worked with countless athletes who would regularly suffer from colds and flus during the winter months and once we increased their carbohydrate intake after their hardest sessions, we saw an improvement in their immune function almost overnight. This is also the case when fat loss is one of your primary goals. As long as you adjust your fat intake and overall calories, considering your body is like a 'sponge' soaking up all the nutrients and calories after these particularly hard sessions, you can still lose body fat, fully recover from workouts and potentially stop yourself getting training-induced colds and flus.

Minimising colds and flus

Staying healthy and injury-free is a key goal for every athlete. You can't work on improving your shooting or passing if you're injured or get stronger and faster if you're in bed with a cold or flu. If you want to perform at your best, you need consistent training and not scattered periods where you're on a physio table or curled up in bed for days at a time. One of the many upsides of training hard is that it helps you get stronger, fitter and faster so that you have a mental and physical edge over your opponents. However, on the flip side, hard training imposes a lot of stress on your immune system, ligaments, tendons and bones. This is why your post-workout meal and the 24-hour post-workout recovery window are so vitally important. I'm not a doctor, and the concept of the immune system supporting nutrition recovery is currently quite underdeveloped in sports science. Thus, there are no absolute rules pertaining to this. However, there are two general guidelines that have worked tremendously well with my athletes over the years and I'll share them below in the hopes that they help you too.

1.   Carbohydrates: Your immune system works best when it has carbohydrates available to it. The only real

job carbohydrates have is to give your body energy and, as I mentioned earlier, there are no essential carbohydrates – the majority of the population could potentially live perfectly healthy lives without consuming another carbohydrate ever again. But you're not like the general population. You're an athlete. Some of the first things I tell any of my athletes to do when they do actually fall sick is to focus on getting rest (no training), sleep (to recover) and increase their carbohydrate intake to help give their body the energy it requires to fight a cold or a mild flu.

However, this is when you are already sick, and as Benjamin Franklin said, 'An ounce of prevention is worth a pound of cure.' Generally, strenuous exercise supresses immune function and provides viruses with a 'window of opportunity' after a workout. This is when you're the most susceptible to attack. I love the old saying, 'You don't get a cold or flu, a cold or flu gets you!' When your immune system is weak, you render yourself vulnerable to falling sick. Making sure you're well-fuelled before, during and after a session helps keep your immune system strong even when everyone else around you is picking up colds and flus.

2.   Time: Have you ever rushed to training straight after work, having completely forgotten to eat your pre-workout meal or dinner? Or have you ever finished a gruelling session only to wait an hour before you getting home and eating your post-workout meal? I know I've done it countless times. If you don't have adequate fuel, your immune system can suffer. This is why it's so important to have your pre-, intra- and post-workout nutrition planned beforehand. The harder the training session, the more important it is to follow your plan rather than leaving it to luck.

3.   Car hack: There are days when you're just not going to be able to stick to, plan or prepare your pre- and post-workout nutrition. One of my hacks with my players is to always have a few scoops of protein and oats (along with some BCAAs) and an empty shaker in your car (or training bag if you don't have a car). This way, even in a worst-case scenario, you have 50 g of oats and a scoop of protein shake before and after training, with BCAAs during, to ensure that you don't compromise your immune system or recovery in general.

Good sources of complete protein, for example, are listed as follows:

- Poultry such as chicken or turkey

- Red meat such as beef or lamb

- Oily or white fish such as salmon, mackerel or cod

- Whey protein powder

- Hemp or rice protein powder

- Eggs

- Cottage cheese

- Greek yoghurt

ALCOHOL

Alcohol and fuelling your body

Carbohydrates, fats and proteins are all capable of providing energy for exercise. Alcohol, however, cannot be used directly by muscles for energy during exercise, no matter how hard you might be working. One of the biggest misconceptions I had when I was in college was that if I continued to train harder, I would just burn through the alcohol in my system and it wouldn't affect my gym or pitch performance. The truth is, this just isn't the case. Only the liver has the specific enzymes needed to break down alcohol. You cannot break it down by training harder either – the liver carries out its job at a fixed speed. I have a little bit of a love-hate relationship with alcohol. I love a glass of wine with a meal or a couple of beers if I'm watching a game, but I hate the feeling that comes with exceeding that amount. My goal here isn't to say alcohol is good or bad but to give you an idea of what's happening to your body when you consume it. You can then decide whether you should factor it into your plan each week.

Why alcohol can halt your progress

Alcohol is metabolised by the liver and, thus, drastically affects your blood sugar balance, particularly when consumed on an empty stomach. This is why you are normally 'starving' after you have five or six alcoholic drinks.

Drinking alcohol, particularly drinks with added sugar, results in a rapid rise in blood sugar. This causes your pancreas to release insulin in an attempt to balance out your blood sugar. Insulin circulates, does what it's supposed to do and then leaves you mildly hypoglycaemic (low blood sugar), ensuring you are excessively hungry after several drinks. Therefore, on top of adding extra calories to your daily intake and causing dehydration, your blood sugar levels are also negatively affected. Thus, the next logical question is, 'Does having alcohol with food minimise its effects?' Not quite, I'm afraid.

Alcohol also works as a 'displacing agent', which means that when you consume alcohol with meals, it serves as a blocking agent and effectively prohibits the absorption of several vitamins and minerals.

Alcohol, fat loss, muscle gain and performance

Now that I've explained how alcohol affects your body, let's take a look at how it affects fat loss, muscle gain and performance on the pitch.

On one hand, your body will not burn body fat or build lean muscle tissue while it's detoxifying itself of alcohol. However, on the other hand, alcohol moves straight to the front of the queue as your primary energy source, which your body will utilise as its 'go to' energy source while it's in your system.

Your body using alcohol as its main energy source is a lot like your car trying to run on water – it will simply break down shortly after you get going. Have you ever gone for a run or a gym session the day after you have had four or five alcoholic drinks, to try and 'sweat' the alcohol out? Additionally, while working out, have you felt like it was coming out through your pores as you trained? That is your body using it as a primary fuel source.

The fact that your body processes alcohol first is the same reason you should avoid it the night before a game. You have to give your liver at least 48 hours to clear out some of the alcohol you have consumed so that your performance on the pitch isn't affected.

How to use

I recommend limiting alcohol to once or twice per week and avoid drinking on the night before games.

Fat loss tip

There are roughly 64 calories in a shot of clear alcohol, vodka and Bacardi for example, and 82 calories in a glass of white wine. Beer has between 200 and 300 calories per pint.

If you want to keep your calories low, limit your alcohol consumption to white wine or clear alcohol and save yourself a fortune in calories.

Comparisons

3 pints of beer: 600-900 kcal

3 glasses of white wine: 246 kcal

3 glasses of vodka and diet mixer: 192 kcal

FAT

When we talk about fat types – saturated, monounsaturated and polyunsaturated – we're actually talking about fatty acids. Fatty acids are chains of carbon and hydrogen atoms attached to a carboxyl group (think of it like a hinge on your bike that keeps individual chains together). Every fat, whether plant or animal, is made up of these same raw materials.

In saturated fat, every link in the fatty acid chain is secured – it's saturated. Monounsaturated fats have just one unsecured link (mono is Latin for 'one'), and polyunsaturated fats have two or more unsecured links in their chains (poly is Latin for 'many').

In truth, almost all the natural fats we eat are a blend of these three kinds of fat. But whatever a fat is mainly made of, whether saturated, monounsaturated or polyunsaturated, we generally refer to it simply as fat. We do the same with macronutrients. Oats, for example, have a little fat and some protein but are primarily comprised of carbohydrates, which is why they are labelled as a 'carbohydrate' food.

Why do we need fat?

- For brain function: Omega 3, for example, plays a critical role in brain function and is crucial for improving decision-making processes on the pitch.

- To burn body fat: Certain types of fats, such as conjugated linoleic acid (CLA), are found in grass-fed cows and pasteurised butter can actually help your body burn fat.

- For steady energy: Fat is the most concentrated source of energy. It can provide you with steady energy throughout the day and keep your blood sugar levels stable.

- To absorb certain vitamins: Vitamins A, D, E, K and carotenoids are all fat soluble i.e. you need to consume them with fat in order to absorb them.

Eating the right kind of fat is absolutely vital for optimal health and physical performance.

Calories and fat

Having an idea of your calorie consumption is important for your fitness goals. If you want to lose weight and your calorie maintenance (the number of calories you need to eat to stay the same weight) is 2,000 kcals, you will probably not lose weight or body fat too quickly if you eat 6,000 kcals every day. On the other hand, if you are trying to build muscle and your maintenance is 2,000 kcals, you need to eat significantly more in order to build lean muscle. However, the amount obviously depends on the speed of your metabolism, current body fat levels and your training program (pitch and gym) in general.

Fat has more calories per gram (9 kcal) than carbs or protein (both 4 kcal). However, the reality is that 500 kcal from fat are absorbed very differently than 500 kcal from carbohydrates. Fat is more satiating, meaning it will leave you feeling fuller for longer, and including good quality fats that help stabilise blood sugar and hunger levels can be the key to losing body fat or building more muscle and giving you steady energy throughout the day.

Not all fat is created equal

One of the biggest misconceptions that I fell victim to in my early twenties was, 'Eating fat will make you fat.' I think a more accurate rephrasing would be, 'Certain fat will make you fat.' The three main types of fat that are important to understand are omega 6, omega 3 and trans fatty acids.

Omega 3 and omega 6

Both essential fatty acids (EFA), omega 3 and omega 6 are considered vital and beneficial. However, omega 3 is normally considered slightly more important, as the modern western diet is likely to be more deficient in omega 3 than omega 6. This is because the king of the omega 3 family, alpha-linolenic acid (ALA), and his metabolically active prince and princess, eicosapentaenoic acid (EPA) and docosahexaenoic acid (DHA), are more unsaturated and prone to damage during cooking and food processing. In other sections of the book, I've spoken about how food processing removes a lot of nutrients from food, and omega 3 is a primary example of this.

Why do I need omega 3?

Omega 3 is actively involved in critical biological functions such as improving cognitive abilities, helping you retain information better, helping you perform complicated tasks more effectively, alleviating pain and inflammation as well as improving insulin sensitivity.

If you find that you have brain fog, pain from inflammation or have body fat to lose, it might be worth increasing your omega 3 intake by including more foods like salmon, flax or chia seeds.

The best sources of omega 3

The best seed oils for omega 3 are flax (also known as linseed), hemp and pumpkin. For example, one of my favourite health shakes includes a mixture of rice or whey protein, flaxseed oil, hemp and pumpkin seeds.

If you eat carnivorous fish, such as mackerel, herring, tuna and salmon, or their oils, you can bypass the conversion stage of alpha linoleic acid and go straight to EPA and DHA. This is why fish-eating cultures (the Japanese culture for example) have three times the omega 3 than their western counterparts. Vegans who eat more seeds tend to have much higher levels of omega 3 as well.

What are the best sources of fat?

- Oily fish such as salmon and mackerel
- Nuts such as almonds, walnuts, or cashews

- Seeds such as pumpkin, linseed or chia
- Oils (flaxseed, hemp)

Again, these are just some of my favourites. Feel free to experiment with other types of fat. However, there is one type of fat that you do need to watch out for.

Avoid this type of fat or you will get fat

Trans-fatty acids or 'trans fats' definition:

'An unsaturated fatty acid of a type occurring in margarines and manufactured cooking oils as a result of the hydrogenations process. Consumption of such acids is thought to increase the risk of atherosclerosis (a disease of the arteries)' – Webster Dictionary.

Trans fats are created as a result of the partial hydrogenation process or, as author of *Eat the Yolks* Liz Wolfe describes it, 'the process of beating an already unhealthy oil into partially hydrogenated submission'. This basically means they convert already unhealthy oils into something even worse! Not only have trans fats been shown to lead to a range of health problems (heart disease, obesity, etc.), but they are also the single worst types of fats if you are trying to reduce your own levels of body fat. Your body can store them pretty easily.

Trans fats normally increase the body fat around your lower abdomen or go to your 'stubborn' areas – the places you struggle to remove body fat from. Not only that but studies have shown that trans fatty acids have a significant impact on your natural level of testosterone as well, entailing that the more trans fats you consume, the less natural testosterone you will produce.

'Trans' is Latin for the opposite side, and hence the name trans fats. Your body doesn't recognise trans fats – their actual chemical makeup is completely foreign to it. Because of this, as soon as you consume them, your body panics and tends to shuttle them straight into the fat pockets or visceral fat (fat over the organs) so as to not damage your vital organs.

This is basically a survival safety mechanism. Your vital organs are safe if the 'unknown' foods – trans fats in this case – are safely tucked away into your fat pockets.

The easiest way to avoid trans fats is to reduce or eliminate deep fat fried or fast food along with certain margarines. Not only will you feel a substantial increase in energy levels but also your process of reducing unwanted body fat will also significant y speed up. Additionally, if you're male, you'll keep your natural testosterone levels elevated.

TESTOSTERONE

Low testosterone and body fat (for the guys)

This next section is mainly for the guys. However, feel free to read it regardless of gender, as there may be something here that could be applicable to your boyfriend, husband or partner.

In some cases, if you are holding a lot of body fat around your hips, stomach and lower back, it can sometimes be an indicator of low testosterone. Belly fat and low testosterone is a bit of a 'chicken or egg' situation. Some studies suggest that low testosterone causes excess belly fat while others claim that excess belly fat contributes to lower levels of testosterone. While the answer is not perfectly clear, the one thing that is clear is that there is obviously a link between the two.

According to the National Institute of Health, testosterone is a sex hormone that plays important roles in the body. In men, it's thought to regulate the sex drive (libido), bone mass, fat distribution, muscle mass and strength, and the production of red blood cells and sperm. Some guys naturally have lower levels of testosterone and others often produce less testosterone as they age.

Nutrition and testosterone

A healthy and balanced diet is crucial if you're looking to optimise natural testosterone production. It's very important to minimise processed foods and use wholefoods for your carb loads.

Also important in producing testosterone is the consumption of both unsaturated and saturated fats as well as cholesterol. Yeah, I said cholesterol. Remember, consumption of dietary cholesterol is extremely different from blood cholesterol (LDL/HDL), and consuming a healthy amount of cholesterol from oysters, free-range eggs, and various other foods is required for producing sex hormones such as testosterone. Believe it or not, cholesterol is the building block of all sex hormones, including testosterone, and your body can't produce testosterone without it.

Last but not least, don't forget to eat plenty of lean protein from lean meats, fish, and organic milk. If you're vegetarian, try to eat plenty of black beans, wild and brown rice and high-protein fruits/veggies like avocados, goji berries, hemp and chia seeds. The key is balance, and higher testosterone comes along with a balanced diet rich in all macronutrients.

Later, I will talk about some of the best natural testosterone-booster supplements for an athlete, but the main way to ramp up testosterone is to avoid processed foods, minimise alcohol intake to once or twice a week (maximum) and get seven to nine hours of sleep every night. The supplements will 'supplement' what you're missing, but nothing beats the basics for bringing it up naturally. I've had guys from the age of 21 (with genetically low testosterone) to males aged 35+ (in whom it lowered with age) all ramp up their sex drive, lower their body fat and improve their mood and energy levels by eating more whole foods, cutting back on alcohol, getting quality sleep (see sleep section for more information on this) and then adding in a few supplements to top it off.

Four low-testosterone quick fixes

1. <u>Testosterone-boosting superfoods:</u> Building your nutritional plan with good quality whole foods, such as complex carbohydrates, healthy fats and complete

proteins, is key. However, if you need an extra 'kick', it might be worth factoring in some of these super foods into your plan.

Oysters: Rich in zinc and protein, oysters have been known to support health and sexual well-being for centuries. Personally, I'm not a massive fan, but I've had several men (and women) explain how their libido increases after the consumption of oysters. Zinc is a precursor for testosterone, so these are a real super food in that context.

Organic Free-Range Eggs: These are rich in healthy fats, cholesterol and highly bio-available albumin protein, which means they are absorbed very effectively. Eggs contain all the building blocks of testosterone and help repair muscle as well as any other naturally ingested protein. This is one food I never mind spending the extra money on.

Garlic: Garlic is rich in allicin and is shown to improve blood flow. Garlic also naturally reduces LDL cholesterol, meaning more good cholesterol available for testosterone production. It's also incredible at staving off colds and flus. So, if you have a lot of games or pre-season in the wet and cold months, this can stop you from getting sick.

Chocolate: Known for centuries to be a natural aphrodisiac, chocolate contains high levels of magnesium, which can regulate estrogen levels. Aim for 85% dark chocolate or raw cocoa if you can.

Broccoli and Cabbage: Both of these contain indole-3-carbinol, which has shown to reduce estrogen levels and, in return, raise testosterone.

Avocados: These are high in vitamin B6, folic acid and have plenty of healthy monounsaturated fats to send your testosterone levels soaring through the roof.

Almonds: Almonds are full of the building blocks of testosterone. Eat them every day if you can. They are also a great food choice for dieters as well as for people looking to add lean muscle. These are probably my favourite 'go to' snack at work or when I travel.

Organic Beef: Grass-fed (if you're living outside of Ireland or the UK) and organic beef is preferred as often as possible. Organic beef is loaded with amino acids, zinc, natural creatine and saturated fats that promote optimal levels of testosterone.

2.   Cut back on alcohol for a few weeks: If you read anything about testosterone, you will see the common trend of 'alcohol is the enemy of testosterone', 'beer kills your sex drive' or some variation of this

description. Granted, it's definitely not ideal for testosterone levels, but the real negative effects come mainly if large doses are consumed. I've talked about this in the alcohol section and, while true that alcohol has been shown to decrease testosterone levels, other ingredients play a role as well. Before you get too worried, I want to stress that moderate alcohol consumption is unlikely to destroy your testosterone levels and is only associated with only a slight decrease in testosterone. In this context, moderate consumption is defined as about 2-3 glasses of wine or bottles of beer on two or three nights during the week.

In fact, both light and moderate alcohol consumption seem to have a variety of health benefits, including reduced heart failure risk, reduced heart attack risk, reduced stroke risk, reduced dementia risk, reduced diabetes risk, etc., and a little bit of alcohol each week is probably fine – just don't overdo it. My advice would be to minimise it for a few weeks until you get your testosterone, body composition and performance on the pitch to a level that you're happy with and then re-introduce it in your nutritional plan.

Exactly how alcohol lowers testosterone is a bit strange, and it takes place on several levels.

So, how *does* alcohol lower testosterone?

The answer varies depending on the type of alcohol you drink. It also varies greatly between the sexes as well.

Beer, for instance, often contains two chemicals that can increase estrogen (and therefore decrease testosterone): phytoestrogen and prolactin. These chemicals are found in hops as well as in barley, two very common ingredients in many beers. Wine also contains phytoestrogen (a chemical contained in many plants), and even some liquors (such as bourbon) contain these chemicals. These chemicals can increase a man's natural levels of estrogen, thereby reducing his testosterone levels.

The added calories from too many beers also cause men to gain weight, and fat has a nasty tendency to produce even more estrogen. But it doesn't end there. For men, ethanol alcohol is a testicular toxin, and we've known for decades that, in large doses, it reduces testosterone function, sperm count, fertility, and can even damage the testes. In fact, alcoholic men often suffer from infertility and abnormally low testosterone. It's funny because women actually have the opposite problem – excessive alcohol consumption often leads to increased testosterone levels – sometimes even resulting in the loss of female sexual characteristics.

The take-home message is that too much alcohol plays havoc with your body's ability to produce hormones correctly, no matter your sex.

So, does alcohol lower testosterone? Yes, but if you control your consumption, you don't really have anything to worry about. Whether you factor it into your program comes down to your personal preference and goals.

3: Sleep

A 2011 study published in the Journal of the American Medical Association (JAMA) reported on the effect of one week of sleep restriction in healthy, young men. Previous studies have shown that a gradual decrease in sleep time is partially responsible for low testosterone in older men.

In the JAMA study, 10 men volunteered to have their testosterone levels checked during eight nights of sleep restriction. They were only allowed five hours of sleep per night. The study found that their daytime testosterone levels decreased by 10-15%. The lowest testosterone levels were seen in the afternoon and evening. The study also found a progressive loss of energy over the week of sleep deprivation. How to maximise your recovery by focusing on high-quality sleep strategies is discussed further in the sleep section of the book.

4: <u>Supplements:</u> When it comes to dietary supplements that boost natural testosterone, you'll stumble across a multitude of options, all making a storm of various claims. Most are absolutely ridiculous and don't really increase anything except for the amount of cash in the pocket of the seller, but there are some that work great for increasing testosterone naturally and won't break the bank.

It's crucial to understand the difference between these products and pick the one that's right for you. Considering all the testosterone-boosting supplements on the market, you can categorise them into two basic groups – the first being testosterone-boosting blends and the second being single and standalone supplements. Personally, I would always opt for the single and standalone supplements, as you know exactly what you're getting and in what amount. Most testosterone-boosting blends are proprietary blends that contain synergistic mixes of vitamins, minerals and herbs that seek to raise testosterone levels naturally. Moreover, although most of these contain well-researched ingredients, they are normally significantly higher in price and can cost you a lot even for a month's supply. With single-ingredient testosterone-boosting supplements, you can purchase more of a single ingredient at a lower price and make your own testosterone-boosting combos at home This allows you to save money and have more of the ingredients that you feel work best for you. Below, you'll find a detailed list of my favourite natural testosterone-boosting supplements that I use myself and recommend to my athletes.

Note: As these are single ingredients, the brand doesn't matter too much. The main thing to look at is the ingredient list for the correct dosage and to make sure there's nothing else added to the product (i.e. filler ingredients).

D-Aspartic Acid: D-Aspartic Acid plays a pivotal role in the manufacturing process of testosterone. Studies have shown that 3 g of D-Aspartic Acic a day can boost testosterone levels by as much as 33% in as little as 12 days. I have found that going up as high as 3 g twice per day when your training schedule is particularly hectic also works great.

ZMA: A combination of zinc, magnesium and vitamin B6 conveniently combined to provide proven results in terms of natural testosterone production. Take the recommend dosage at night time on an empty stomach with a glass of water for best results.

Resveratrol: Shown to reduce estrogen levels, which in turn boosts testosterone through natural feedback loops.

Horny Goat Weed (Epimedium extract): A popular aphrodisiac that combines nicely with other natural testosterone boosters.

Maca Root: Used for energy, stamina, and has adaptogenic properties (helps your body resist the damaging effects of stress). I add 5–10g of organic maca root powder to my daily smoothie.

Below is a very basic sample diet for a male athlete (females can half the amount of food). Of course, it is always better to have a nutritional plan that's designed around your particular goals, and although I have all the macronutrient and calorie calculations calculated for the players that I work with in my programs, this should serve to provide a good picture of how to space your meals and time them throughout the day.

Breakfast:	**8:00am**: 70 g of porridge oats and two free-range organic eggs or 2-4 oat protein pancakes (recipe below)
Morning Snack:	**11:00am:** 120 g of Greek yoghurt and 2 teaspoons of pumpkin seeds or overnight on-the-go protein oats
Lunch:	**2:00pm:** Salmon or steak with unlimited broccoli and 300 g of baby new potatoes or a wholegrain bread sandwich with chicken or tuna.
Pre-training snack:	**5:00pm**: Three handful of almonds and 1 scoop of protein
Dinner or post workout:	**8:00pm:** Sweet potato shepherd's pie (recipe below)
Before bed snack (optional):	**10:30pm:** 150g of cottage cheese or a peanut butter and berry protein smoothie (recipe below)

Note: I would try to limit your protein supplement to one or two servings per day. This includes adding it to other recipes i.e. protein pancakes, on-the-go protein oats and peanut butter and berry protein smoothies. For more recipes, check out my programs and/or social media channels by searching Brian Keane Fitness.

Oat protein pancakes recipe:

Ingredients:

- 1 whole egg
- 1 egg white
- 120 ml of unsweetened almond milk
- 25 g or 1 scoop of whey
- 60 g scoop of oats
- ½ tablespoon of cinnamon
- Stevia drops/1 teaspoon vanilla extract

Instructions:

1. Blend your eggs and add the rest of the ingredients. Set your pan to a low/medium heat and spray liberally with 1 cal cooking spray.

2. Add about 4-6 tablespoons of the batter (depending on your size of pan), fry it for about 1-2 minutes on first side, flip, then fry for about 10 seconds or until you can comfortably move it around in the pan.

3. Repeat process for the remaining batter.

Calories Per Batch (four pancakes)	Carbohydrate	Protein	Fats
430	45 g	40 g	10 g

Sweet potato shepherd's pie

Ingredients:

- 600 g, sweet potato, raw
- 400 g, uncooked minced lamb or lean beef
- 300 ml stock, beef, homemade
- 1 onion
- 1 medium carrot, raw
- 4 cloves of garlic, raw
- 2 tbsp of tomato puree
- 1 tbsp of coconut oil
- 200 g of red kidney beans

Instructions:

1. Boil the kettle and cook/steam your sweet potato for 15-20 minutes. Finely chop the onion and garlic, then add to a frying pan with the coconut oil and cook until they become soft and golden in colour.

2. Add the lamb or lean beef mince and cook until all the pinkness has gone. Add the beef stock and stir, then simmer for 5 minutes. Add your kidney beans to the mince. Chop the carrot and add it. Finally, add the tomato puree and stir the mixture. Transfer it to a pie dish.

3. Strain your sweet potato and mash until smooth. Then cover the mince with it and pop in the oven on 200 degrees C for 30 minutes until cooked.

Calories Per Batch	Carbohydrate	Protein	Fats
1,920	190 g	115 g	67 g
Calories for 1 person (making 4)	Carbohydrate	Protein	Fats
450	47 g	29 g	16 g

Tip: This is a big dish, so an option is to have one serving for dinner and then put the left overs in the fridge to have as lunch for the next few days.

Peanut butter and berry protein smoothie

Ingredients:

- 1 scoop or 25 g vanilla whey protein
- 250 ml of almond milk (unsweetened)
- 1 tbsp of natural peanut butter
- 1 drop of organic stevia
- ¼ cup of raspberries
- ¼ cup of black or blueberries
- 1 cup of ice

Instructions:

1. Put it all into a blender and blend. Add ice or water for desired texture.

Calories Per Smoothie	Carbohydrate	Protein	Fats
350	38 g	30 g	9 g

CHAPTER 2:

SUPPLEMENTS

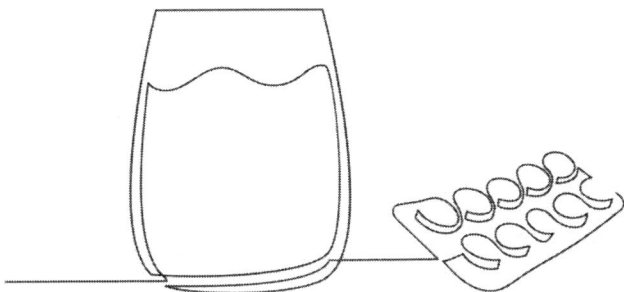

The golden supplement rules for athletes

Certain supplements can work incredibly well for athletes. They can help speed up your recovery, support your immune system (so you don't get sick) as well as help make you stronger and faster. However, they will NOT replace the fundamentals of a good training and nutritional program. You can take the best supplements in the world, but if you skip the other two, you're going to see very minimal improvement.

As you'll see in the training section of the book, your workouts should be focused on improving performance by incorporating hypertrophy, strength and metabolic conditioning along with a good nutritional plan based on carb cycling and eating high-quality nutrient-dense food. Once you have both of these in place, the right supplements can have a much greater impact on your performance.

Again, the supplement list for players I work with directly varies depending on each person's specific goals, but there are a few best practices and supplements that work for most athletes regardless of their goal or gender. When taken at the right times and in the correct dosage, they can speed up recovery and help with fat loss or muscle building in combination with your nutritional plan.

Before I get into which supplements work, there are two points I want to touch on. Personally, I was fooled into spending lots of money on useless supplements because of a couple of misconceptions that I held. I have shared them with you below.

1) You need a fat burner to get lean or ripped and

2) You need a weight gainer to get muscular and jacked (and worse, you need both to get muscular AND ripped.).

I regularly talk on my GAA Lean Body Podcast about how I was fooled (for years) into buying every supplement that was advertised with my favourite fitness models, influencers or sports people. I thought, *Well, if I use that supplement, I'll look like them* – so, month after month, I would pool together the last bits of my college beer money and go buy the new 'silver bullet' supplement.

Month after month, the changes would be so minimal (and the cost so maximal) that I got very disheartened and started to do my own research on supplements. Eight years later, I'm actually a bigger fan of supplements now than I was back then; the difference is I know now **which** ones to use and **how** to use them.

I've saved hundreds and probably thousands at this stage by focusing on using the fundamental supplements that work for me and avoid the latest 'fat-burner ripped fuel sliced abs 6000' or 'muscular enhancer weight gainer 5 million' – of course, these are not real products, but a quick Google search will show you some of the most ridiculous names given to fat burning and weight gaining supplements

Now that you have some background, I can present my golden supplement rules for athletes:

Golden Rule #1: Avoid over-the-counter fat burners

To really cement my point, I have to say that most over-the-counter fat burners work 100% in the short-term – 'short-term' being the operative word here.

A good over-the-counter fat burner will provide you with more energy and possibly reduce your appetite. Most over-the-counter fat burners run off different receptors in your body, but as anyone who drinks three cups of coffee a day can attest to, you build up a tolerance to the stimulant effects pretty quickly. So, even though the fat burner was giving you energy and the caffeine was probably helping you release fat from the cells initially as well, once your receptors become downregulated (i.e. you develop a caffeine tolerance), the fat burner will stop giving you that energy and will effectively stop having any effect on your body. This means that the 'fat-burning supplement' has now just turned into a really expensive cup of coffee.

Just to clarify, I'm not actually against fat burners; some of them, such as green tea extract, caffeine by itself and l-carnitine tartrate, can really help support your fat loss goals without all the negative side effects. I'm talking about the proprietary-blend fat burners with multiple ingredients and fillers that are sold as a 'quick fix'.

However, my biggest issue with fat burners is probably the known 'rebound' that occurs for most people post-use. It's not uncommon to lose body fat and weight* using a fat burner; however, to keep it off when you stop using it is another matter entirely.

Note: Although mentioned earlier, it's worth reiterating it here – 'losing weight' and 'losing body fat' is not the same thing. Losing weight is reducing numbers on a scale, while losing body fat is losing fat off your body. In some instances, you will get both i.e. the numbers on the scale will reduce along with the fat on your body, but not in every case.

Most fat burners have time-released stimulants that supply consistent energy to you throughout the day, replacing food. This is great while you are using them; you have more energy, don't need food to function and are more alert throughout the day but, alas, what goes up must come down.

I'll never forget this one experience I had with an extremely strong over-the-counter fat burner when I was still in college. I took this fat burner in the morning and went to the gym for three hours. That same evening, I played over three hours of seven-a-side soccer. All I had eaten that entire day was an apple. A single apple! I woke up the next day feeling like I had been run down by a truck. During my six hours of training and a full day of college, I never stopped to question where the energy was coming from, but I certainly felt it the following day. This story should give you an idea of the strength of some of the over-the-counter fat burners. I bought this particular brand (which has been banned since) from the local health store where I bought my porridge. Remember, just because you can buy them over-the-counter does not automatically make them safe or healthy.

Because fat burners keep your body in a consistent state of 'fight or flight', your entire recovery and hormonal system can become compromised. If you have ever used a fat burner and got up to the use the toilet in the middle of the night only to find yourself wide awake as soon as you climb back into your bed, it's usually due to the over-activation of this 'fight or flight' response and the cortisol circulating in your body.

When you wake up, your body spikes cortisol, which is actually the natural way to wake up. However, with the presence of excess stimulants in your system and overworking of your adrenals, this process can become massively heightened i.e. it's 3 a.m., you wake and your body thinks it's ready to start the day. So, a lot of over-the-counter fat burners can negatively affect your sleep, and you'll see the importance of getting high-quality sleep when it comes to building muscle, losing fat or improving performance and recovery later on in the book. But what causes the rebound then?

Generally, there are two main causes for the rebound:

1.   Energy crash and poor food choices: When you stop taking your fat burner, you generally come out of that state of 'fight or flight'. This was giving you consistent, albeit 'short term', energy, leaving you with an incredible drop or reduction in energy upon discontinuing its use. What do you tend to reach for

when your energy is at an all-time low? You got it – food. Additionally, it's normally not broccoli, porridge or chicken either. When that ultimate energy low hits, you tend to reach for sugars, chocolate, biscuits, cakes or other stimulant drinks. From a basic calories in – calories out standpoint, this overconsumption of food can lead to that dreaded 'rebound'. A rebound is normally the term used for when you look and feel worse than you did when you initially started taking the fat burner. This doesn't even account for the hormonal disruption that can occur due to this unnatural extended period of caloric restriction.

2.   <u>Your appetite can become uncontrollable:</u> Most over-the-counter fat burners normally include strong 'appetite suppressant' ingredients and, as the name suggests, these suppress your appetite.

That's fine while you are taking them, but think about what happens when you come off them after your appetite has been supressed for 6-8 weeks? I like to think of it like pulling back a rubber band; the harder and further you pull it back (suppressed appetite), the harder it will snap back.

A couple of days after the experience I mentioned above, I was utterly ravenous! I must have consumed 10,000-

12,000kcals two days later. It also doesn't take a rocket scientist to figure out that if I was trying to lose body fat, consuming 100 kcals one day and 12,000 kcals on the other is probably not going to support me all that much.

This is what over-the-counter fat burners can do. As I mentioned, just because you can buy it from a local shop* doesn't deem it good or safe for you. I can go to any fast-food restaurant and buy cheeseburgers every day of the week, that doesn't make it good for me. We have an availability bias in our brain; it's one of the cognitive biases that has evolved over thousands of years and makes us think that because it's available, it must be 'okay'. Remember, not too long ago, you could buy opium on the open market (heroin is derived from the morphine alkaloid found in opium), so don't ever use something just because you can buy it over the counter.

Side note: A lot of over-the-counter fat burners (and some pre-workouts) aren't FDA approved either, and some top inter-county players have been banned due to certain ingredients contained in these supplements. Just be careful when choosing your supplements. If you don't understand the ingredients in it, ask an expert or do your own research on what you can and cannot use as an athlete.

I must have experimented with every fat burner on the market from the age of nineteen to twenty-three and have experienced all the positive and negative effects that came with them. One of my favourite quotes, which closed out my first book *The Fitness Mindset*, was,

'*Smart people learn from their mistakes; really smart people learn from other people's mistakes.*' – Brandon Mull

The key to losing fat is to find a good nutritional plan based around your goals along with a training program that syncs with it. There are fat burners, such as green tea extract and l-carnitine, that won't have a negative effect on you mentally, physically or physiologically. But I promise you, if you lose fat the right way, you will lose it, keep it off and your performance on the pitch won't suffer either!

The most important supplements for athletes

For athletes, it's all about recovery. There are some great supplements that will help make you stronger in the gym, such as creatine, which can translate into improved strength on the pitch, and beta alanine, which can help buffer lactic acid and prevent that massive build-up during training and gym sessions or during games. However, in most cases, the difference between good and the great players comes down to their ability to recover between games, workouts and training sessions.

The better your recovery, the higher level of output you can put out each time. Think about it this way, who would you rather play against – a person who trains on the pitch twice a week and plays a game on the weekend or a person who does that PLUS another three or four gym sessions that are focused on activating and 'firing' their glutes to make them faster, metabolic conditioning to make them aerobically fitter and core work to break through tackles more effectively? I know which one I'd prefer to play against.

The reality is, when following the right program, effort = results. We see it time and time again at inter-county levels; the top players are rarely the ones with the most natural talent – they are the ones that put in the most work and recover better than everyone else. You may not want to necessarily play at that level; but when your nutrition is in alignment with your specific goals, supplements have the ability to enhance recovery even further, which can potentially elevate you to the next level and alter your body composition faster.

Post-workout recovery is crucial

Nutrition is always going to be number one here. You want to replenish glycogen stores (carb stores) as soon as you finish any intense session so that you are not running on empty (fat stores) in the following day's session. The two supplements you may consider adding to your post-workout regimen (pitch and gym) are a good, absorbable whey protein and/or BCAAs.

Again, depending on each individual's goals, your supplement requirements will be different. For example, if muscle building is your primary goal, you may add creatine and better alanine before and/or after your workout, or you can possibly add green tea extract or l-carnitine tartrate if fat loss is the goal. However, I'll list some of my personal favourites below, which can work great for nearly any athlete.

1. *Whey protein*

The numerous benefits of whey protein include increase in muscular strength and size, decrease in body fat and a faster recovery time.

Muscle protein synthesis is a scientific phrase thrown around a lot, which basically means that this synthesis enables muscle growth and is an important process involved in increasing muscle size and strength.

Resistance training alone can increase rates of protein synthesis. However, it also increases rates of protein breakdown. For muscle growth to occur, you need to tip the scale in favour of protein synthesis while trying to minimise breakdown.

Consuming whey protein after workouts can substantially increase muscle protein synthesis. Whey protein is a fast-digesting protein that enters the bloodstream rapidly. This allows it to get to your muscles faster and create a bigger spike in protein synthesis as compared to food sources.

Dosage: The amount you use can vary depending on your body weight and protein requirements, but 25-50 g per serving for men and 10-25 g per serving for women thirty minutes after exercise is a good place to start.

2.   *Branch Chain Amino Acids (BCAAs)*

BCAAs are made up of three essential amino acids – leucine, isoleucine and valine. They are essential because the body is unable to produce them using other amino acids and they have to be ingested through food or supplements.

A large percentage of dietary amino acids are oxidised and wasted even before reaching the circulatory system. The exceptions to this pattern are the BCAAs. Over 80% of the dietary content of leucine, valine and isoleucine reaches circulation.

Whey protein is naturally high in BCAAs, but adding another 3-10 g depending on your bodyweight before, during or after your workouts can improve your recovery further. Again, it depends on your overall nutrition. If you are consuming enough high-quality protein in your main meals, you may not need any extra BCAAs.

Dosage: The dose varies depending on your bodyweight and training program, but a good starting point is 5-10 g before or after a workout for men and 3-5 g for women.

3. Caffeine

Caffeine is a staple ingredient in many popular fat-burning and pre-workout supplements. It primarily helps you lose body fat in two ways:

1) By boosting your metabolism: Ingesting caffeine jump-starts the process of lipolysis, which occurs when your body releases free fatty acids into the bloodstream to be used for energy. In other words, caffeine boosts your metabolism and can help you burn fat.

2) By giving you an energy boost: If there's one thing that everyone knows about coffee and caffeinated drinks or pills, it's that caffeine is quite a strong stimulant. It increases alertness and wards off drowsiness temporarily, which means you can perform certain tasks more efficiently or for longer on caffeine.

This applies for physical tasks as well as mental tasks. It entails that a little shot of caffeine can give you the energy you need to give 100% during games or workouts. Further, giving 100% in the gym or on the pitch means you'll get the results you want faster.

Dosage: If you don't regularly ingest a lot of caffeine, a couple hundred milligrams or a strong cup of black coffee will likely produce noticeable effects. You may want to start with 100 mg to see how it goes and then up your intake to 200 mg. You can then increase the dose by 50 mg if you're still not experiencing any effects. Do be careful to not overdo it, as the side effects of a caffeine overdose can range from anxiety and insomnia to death.

Take it thirty minutes before your workout to release free fatty acids to be burnt while you train and to increase physical and mental alertness for games. However, be aware that caffeine has just over a five-hour half-life. If you take it too late at night, it can negatively affect your sleep. This means that if you consume 200 mg of caffeine at 12 p.m., 100 mg will still be in your system at 5 p.m.

How to make your own weight-gainer shake

I have one other massive 'pet peeve' with supplements and it's weight gainers.

Just to argue both sides, weight gainers definitely serve a purpose if you're looking to add size. The message is pretty good; you need to eat more calories than you burn and weight gainers can give you extra calories.

However, to get those calories from weight gainers alone is probably the single biggest waste of money when it comes to supplements. Most weight gainers have small servings that average between 500-1,000 kcal per serving. They're normally a mixture of protein and maltodextrin or some other cheap or low-quality carbohydrate and retail at €50 or more.

As someone who has been in the fitness industry for a long time, I'm telling you now that the €50 tub you are buying probably cost a tenth of that to make at scale. If you were to buy those ingredients separately, you would save yourself an absolute fortune!*

Side note: If you are someone who has a well-paying job where you really struggle with time, then over-the-counter weight gainers can be more convenient. You can leave them at work or in your car, so you always have a source of calories at hand. In such a scenario, they definitely serve a purpose.

Personally, I'm not a big fan of the ingredients used in most weight-gaining shakes either. I prefer to use more nutrient-dense ingredients and make my own homemade weight gainer. You get all the benefits of the calories and improved absorption at a tenth of the cost. I have put one of my recipes for a weight-gainer shake below to give you an idea of the same.

100 g oats

4 tbsp of natural peanut butter

1 tbsp of coconut oil

1 scoop of whey protein

500-1,000 ml of coconut or almond milk

Calories: 1,000kcal

Blend it all together in a shake

This shake has around 1,000 kcals and you can always add an apple, berries or other fruits to it in order to bump up the carbohydrates and increase the number of calories. If you have two of them a day, which is the same dosage recommended for most weight gainers, then you are already at 2,000 kcals before you have had any of your meals. If you really want to 'bulk up', save your money and use it to buy real food. Just add this shake (it's my personal 'easy bulk up shake') and, along with a good nutritional plan, you will find yourself in a calorie surplus rather quickly.

CHAPTER 3:

TRAINING

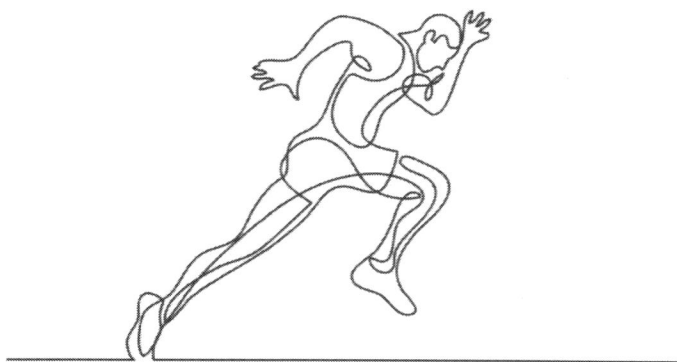

Introduction

How do muscles get bigger? If you lift weights, eat and rest, your muscles grow. While this is fact, the science goes much deeper. It's not as simple as picking up a weight and just moving it from A to B. I spoke in *The Fitness Mindset* about the importance of creating tension on the muscle during workouts, i.e. controlled movements from point A to point B, to elicit the most fibre tears in order to make the muscle grow back bigger and stronger. This is provided you consume enough calories and amino acids from food for your body to perform the repair, of course.

However, as an athlete, there's one more element that needs to be factored in so that you can build lean muscle and not have it affect your performance in a negative way. This element is functionality.

Will having more muscle make me slower?

One of the familiar phrases thrown around during my youth was, 'Lifting weights will make you slower on the pitch,' or, 'If you have to do weights, do them in the off season when it's okay for you to be slower.' Over the years, I've heard countless variations of this. Before I go on, I would like to quash this 'one size fits all' misconception along with playing the devil's advocate for where this misconception probably comes from.

As with most things in life, 'A little knowledge is dangerous.' In the case of weights or resistance training slowing you down, yes, it is physically possible that it could potentially have a negative impact on your speed. If you plan on going into the weights room and just lifting or moving a weight without purpose, along with following a one-size-fits-all squat, bench and deadlift program without any recovery strategy or system for keeping you loose and flexible, then yes, there is a pretty high probability that you will become slower when you go back on the pitch. It's also worth mentioning that this style of training can greatly increase your risk of injury. If you lift weights consistently in just one plane of motion, work with incorrect movement patterns for your sport or load and fatigue your muscles too close to pitch sessions or games, then weights or resistance training can slow you down. So that's that – I suppose lifting weights or using resistance training does make you slower on the pitch? Well, not exactly. On the contrary, following the right training program based on activating your glutes more efficiently and keeping your hip flexors and kinetic chain loose can actually make you faster! Build this into your program with the right nutritional plan and you can actually add lean muscle to your frame or get bigger whilst getting faster at the same time!

The idea that weight training can slow you down was, and obviously still is, a massive misconception. But to be fair, as mentioned above, it can be partially right. Performing certain movements and adding resistance (i.e. lifting weights) in one plane of motion for the wrong rep ranges and parameters can indeed make you slower. If you are doing a barbell squat for three sets of 10 repetitions, followed by three sets of 15 repetitions of leg extensions, followed by a leg press for another three sets of 10 repetitions, it can lead to a whole host of problems in terms of building muscle in movement patterns that don't transfer to the pitch. If you build muscle in one plane of motion, in movement patterns that don't cross over to the pitch, then you are asking for that muscle to pull, strain and even tear. This is exactly what happened to me when I first started lifting. I did it and paid the price.

I started lifting weights in my bedroom at the age of thirteen. I had spent the previous two years doing push-ups and pull-ups in that same room. My parents, both of whom have all the Ireland medals in football and basketball respectively, used to give me £1 for every fifty push-ups I could do without stopping. My local club was and still is a very small parish, so I always played two grades above my age bracket; my coaches always told me that I had to be stronger to be able to keep up with the older boys. There was no restricted-age playing grade when I was younger, so I played under-14 at the age of eleven, under-16 at twelve, minor at thirteen, under-21 at fourteen and made my club senior debut at 15. This definitely helped me build my body and strength quicker than most players my age. As my figurative bar was higher, I was comparing my build, strength and ability to players much older than me. This turned out to be a blessing and a curse, as it led me to weight lifting in my bedroom at age thirteen to try and get bigger and stronger for games. The Internet was only coming along then and I had no way of knowing if I was doing things correctly or not. I continued to lift for three years until my parents finally relented and bought me a gym membership for my 16th birthday. They had their reservations, mostly because they had always been told, 'Weight training stunts your growth.' Up until that point, I even had to hide my dumbbells and barbells in my wardrobe underneath my clothes and lock my bedroom door when I wanted to lift weights after school. Upon retrospection, I'm not sure what my parents thought their fifteen-year-old son was doing in a locked bedroom after school, but I assure you, I was lifting weights...

Does lifting weights stunt your growth?

I also want to add a side note on weight training stunting your growth. Resistance or weight training stunting your growth is a myth. However, similar to 'weights make you slower', it probably has some baseline of truth. Lifting weights incorrectly, especially while you're still growing as a teenager can negatively affect your posture and make you slouch forward; this is particularly true if you consistently load or add resistance to the front of your body i.e. do bench presses and push-ups and don't do the complimentary pulling movements for your back and rear deltoids (the muscle on the back of your shoulders). I had this problem for years, as I would do countless push-ups and bench presses and never any rowing movements or back exercises. This left me with a slouch that took me nearly three years of gym work in my early twenties to correct.

Also, lifting weights incorrectly as a teenager can increase your risk of getting injured. I feel it's worth adding that lifting weights incorrectly can increase the risk of injury for anybody, but teenagers are especially at high risk owing to the fact that their bodies are still growing. That being said, performing the movements or exercises correctly with perfect form hasn't been shown to have any negative effects on growth and can actually increase their strength, speed and power on the pitch.

How the wrong program can really mess you up!

We didn't have a lot of money growing up and even when we did, my parents always made myself and my sister work hard for our money. I got my first job cleaning dishes, pots and pans when I was thirteen. I saved for months and finally bought myself a set of dumbbells so that I could train in my bedroom. I had about ten fitness magazines at this point and imitated every workout that was in them. I didn't understand the difference between muscular strength, muscular endurance, muscular power or even the basic parameters of hypertrophy (tearing fibres in the 8-10 rep range for maximum muscle growth).

I copied the workouts in the magazines and, over the course of about a year, my body composition started to change. Then at sixteen, not only was I allowed to buy a weight bench and a barbell for my bedroom, but my parents bought me a gym membership in the local gym to help me rehabilitate from my first knee dislocation (my first of three dislocations before I turned twenty-one).

I was really in heaven now! I had all the weights and machines I could ever need and was going to change my body to look like the guys on the magazines and be the biggest and strongest guy on the pitch, or so I thought. My dream was to finally move out of the corner- or wing-forward position and into the central positions so I could have more of an impact in games for all the teams I was playing for. I would love to say that, from that day onwards, I got bigger, leaner and stronger and my performance skyrocketed, but that's not what happened. Granted, I did get bigger and stronger and did, as a result, move to the central positions on nearly all my teams, but something really peculiar kept happening. I kept pulling, straining and tearing different muscles. First, my groin would strain, then my hamstring would go a month later and, two months later, I would tear my quad. At the time, I didn't understand how supercompensation worked. It's when one muscle is weak, tight or not activating, the muscles around it tighten and try to compensate for it. For example, if you have ever had one bad injury and were plagued that entire season with niggles and strains elsewhere, it all usually occurs because of that one main injury and the supercompensation principle. I was also extremely tight after every training, gym and pitch session. I felt like an eighty-year-old man after every workout and I had no idea why!

I was in the gym at least three days a week, on the pitch another three or four days a week, eating what I thought was good food and doing all the exercises that were in the magazines; but I was still felt really tight and rigid all the time.

Having since qualified as a strength and conditioning coach and knowing then what I know now, I realise that when you train like a bodybuilder (which is effectively the workouts that were in the magazines at that time and are today's social media workout equivalent), your body builds (hence the name 'bodybuilding'). However, it's rightly not called 'improved performance bodybuilding', and for good reason. They say your mess becomes your message, and I've been fortunate enough to work with hundreds of players who have come through my programs over the years, a lot of whom were going down a similar path I had. It really is a case of knowledge is power while also recognising that a little knowledge can be very dangerous. I knew weights would make me bigger and stronger; but I didn't know that they could also mess me up if I used them incorrectly.

Regardless of your age or starting point, if you're a fifteen-year-old about to pick up your first weight ever, a twenty-four-year-old looking to get onto the county panel or a thirty-one-year-old trying to star on your club team in order to win titles and trophies for your local club, this section, along with the following sections, will hopefully allow you to learn from my mistakes so that you can build your body to the best it has ever been while elevating your pitch performance to new heights.

As I said before, knowledge is power, and understanding the difference between strength, endurance and power can give you a massive advantage when building or following an off-field program.

The difference between strength, endurance and power

Traditionally, strength training can develop three components of muscle fitness – strength, endurance and power. I'm going to add one more to list – composition – which, in this context, is the way the muscle looks.

Growing up, I remember being so frustrated with my coaches when I'd ask them about weight training. Although I always wanted to be bigger, stronger and faster so as to improve my performance on the pitch, I also wanted to look good. I wanted better shape, more muscle and abs as well.

To their credit, the best coaches told me that weight training would indeed improve my performance, make me stronger and potentially make me faster, but it wouldn't necessarily change the way my body looked (traditional strength and conditioning). On the other hand, the personal trainers and competitive bodybuilders that I spoke to told me weight training would make me look better but it wouldn't really improve my sporting performance (traditional bodybuilding).

This was fifteen years ago and, as much as I'd love to

say that GAA is now the leading authority in combining everything in the world of sports performance, nutrition and body composition, this is unfortunately still an issue with a lot of coaches that hold the same beliefs that frustrated me so much fifteen years ago.

One of the reasons I created my GAA Lean Body Program was due to my own frustration of not being able to combine the two. Just to clarify, if you don't care about how you look and just want to improve your sporting performance, then a normal one-rep max Olympic lift style strength and conditioning program can work great. The same applies if you don't care about your performance on the pitch – a standard hypertrophy 8-10 rep range program will work great; but if you are like me and want the best of both worlds, then you need to combine the best of both disciplines.

I love the Gandhi quote, 'Be the change you want to see.' So, instead of giving up on figuring out why there was no way of combining the best of both worlds, I decided to find a way. Having travelled the world as a professional fitness model for two years while studying to become a strength and conditioning coach, I found that you can indeed have the best of both worlds. You just need to make sure that everything in your training is geared towards those specific goals. If you're looking to get bigger, add more muscle to your frame and improve your strength to break into your senior team, then you design your program around that. Alternately, if you're looking to get leaner, build a six pack and become the best player on your club or county team, then you base your entire program around that. You can't hit a target you can't see; but as long as you know what the end target is, you can design a program around it.

For strength, endurance and power, the amount of weight lifted, the speed of movement and the number of repetitions will determine which aspect gets developed the most. In general, using heavy weights for a lower number of repetitions (fewer than 8) develops strength and size, using lighter weights for a higher number of repetitions develops endurance and explosive movements develop power. Add in some hypertrophy (8-10 reps), choose the correct exercise, combine the best of all worlds and before you know it, your body composition AND your performance start to improve synergistically.

Muscular Strength:

Muscular strength is the amount of force a muscle can produce, for example, the amount of weight that can be lifted. Generally, this is thought to be developed by heavy weights (and it is), but what's more important is the overall training parameters that you're working in, your rep ranges, sets and rest. True, you can go and lift as heavy as possible for 5 or 6 repetitions and you will get stronger, but you also increase your risk of injury and thus, your form (discussed below) is essential. Generally, the larger the muscle, the stronger it's thought to be. Although other factors, such as neuromuscular adaptations and the number of fibres controlled and recruited by your nervous system, also affect your strength. We all know that skinny tough guy or girl who is surprisingly strong.

Muscular Endurance:

Muscular endurance is the ability of a muscle to continue contracting against resistance. This is developed by maintaining a constant workload for increasing periods of time – lifting a weight for 12 or more repetitions then building up to say 15 reps, 20 reps and so on as endurance improves. Long distance cycling will develop muscle endurance in the quad muscles, for example. My favourite way to build muscular endurance in order to improve performance on the pitch and stay going in the last 10 minutes when everyone else is getting tired is called 'metabolic conditioning', which I'll discuss in more detail now.

Metabolic Conditioning:

The word 'metabolic conditioning' is thrown around quite a bit in fitness today. In one setting, it may mean something as simple as high-intensity intervals while, in a different gym, it may consist of a complex circuit involving kettle bells, battle ropes and medicine ball work. So what does metabolic conditioning actually mean? Furthermore, what types of metabolic workouts are the most effective for you as an athlete?

Metabolic conditioning simply refers to structured patterns of work and rest periods to elicit a desired response from the body. This desired response is usually to maximise the efficiency of a particular energy system, which is working at maximum capacity or, what some call, an 'all-out sprint' in most cases.

The body has several different methods of getting energy. Different ratios of work-to-rest periods call upon different energy systems and cause specific adaptations. That's why you can be really good at sprints and terrible at long-distance running or doing 'laps' of the pitch – they both require different energy systems.

Researchers in the Journal of Strength and Conditioning Research concluded that a metabolic conditioning workout should be based on desired outcomes and an individual's level of fitness. For instance, a full-back or full-forward looking to add size might have a different work-to-rest ratio than a wing-back or wing-forward looking to get leaner or run farther. Pairing difficult exercises together and blowing through a circuit with no regards to timing isn't nearly as beneficial as a planned attack. If you're an advanced trainer and your goal is to build muscle and improve strength, your workout should be different from a beginner looking to lose body fat and get faster.

To be able to fully apply the concepts of metabolic conditioning, lets first look at the main ways the body gets energy during exercise.

Exercise metabolism: The basics

Metabolism simply refers to how we break down food for energy. Everything we ingest must be broken down into smaller particles in order to be used by our body. This is discussed in greater detail in the nutrition section of the book, but I'll provide a simplified version here for context. There are three primary pathways for metabolism that each has its own place and purpose.

The Immediate System: Phosphagen

Commonly referred to as the creatine phosphate pathway, think of this system as the fastest and most powerful method of obtaining energy. It's mainly utilised when performing power exercises that last less than 10 seconds (20-40 metre sprints for example). More important than the duration is the recovery time. In this system, since it's so quick and powerful, it takes around three to five minutes to fully recover. If you have ever watched a track training session by Usain Bolt or any top Olympic sprinter, you will see that they will go flat out for their nine or ten second sprint and then rest three to five minutes before they do it again. This utilises their creatine phosphate system.

The Intermediate System: Glycolytic

Called the glycolytic pathway, this is an intermediate system that provides energy for activities lasting between one to four minutes. It's primarily used in shorter-duration, intense activities, including weightlifting and mid-distance running intervals (400-800 m). The glycolytic pathway takes between one and three minutes to recover. In the nutrition section of this book, you will see why keeping glycogen stores full or 'carb loading' is so important for athletes.

The Long-Duration System: Aerobic

This long-lasting energy system can keep up with hours upon hours of easy-to-moderate intensity work. Since we have almost limitless amounts of fuel for the aerobic system in the form of fat, it can recover in a matter of seconds. This is the system most marathon runners primarily use.

With the three major pathways outlined, keep in mind that there is always an interplay between the three for athletes. Although phosphagen and glycolytic are the two main players, no one pathway is working at any given time. During a workout, training session or a game, each system can be contributing to some degree; however, certain work-to-rest ratios call upon a particular primary system.

Developing your metabolic conditioning circuit

The purpose of metabolic conditioning is to maximise the efficiency of a particular energy system to perform better on the pitch and help develop your desired physique.

One added benefit is the increase of caloric burn even after the workout is finished. Such high intensity during a training session increases EPOC (excess post-exercise oxygen consumption, informally called afterburn). The measurably increased rate of oxygen intake following strenuous activity leads to a higher resting metabolism for the next few hours according to the Journal of Strength and Conditioning Research. Simply put, after a workout of this type, you are burning more calories even while you are resting.

If your goal was to become better in endurance positions, where you have much more ground to cover, you could be better off incorporating longer circuits with minimal rest in between exercises. Keep in mind that the intensity of the set should remain as high as possible throughout the specified work duration. In order to elicit the desired response, the body must be pushed in terms of performance. I like to use the 1-10 RPE scale (rate of perceived exertion). For example, 1 is how you feel when you roll out of bed in the morning, 5 is a good-paced brisk walk and 10 is a flat-out sprint. If you're supposed to be working at a level 9 or a 10 for your metabolic conditioning circuit and you're still able to hold a conversation with your team or gym mate, you're not working hard enough. You're better off doing three or four minutes of a metabolic conditioning workout where your rate of perceived exertion is at a 10 out of 10 in terms of intensity instead of twenty minutes of floating between 5 and 7.

Here's a quick and simple sample metabolic conditioning workout:

1. Plyometric (clapping) Push-Ups
2. Box Jumps
- 20 reps of each
- 4 sets
- Rest 90 seconds between sets

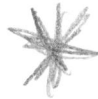

Muscular Power:

Muscular power is the ability to produce both strength and speed. It involves generating a great force as rapidly as possible and is therefore characterised by explosive movements. It is normally developed by lifting near maximal weights (a weight heavy enough to allow 1-5 repetitions) very rapidly and is traditionally an important aspect of performance for most sports. However, the key for building muscular power and improving the shape and size of the muscle for body composition is manipulating the tempo (the speed at which you move the weight up and down) from the muscular power parameter and combining it with the rep range parameters from hypertrophy. This can also reduce the risk of injury, as you're not lifting incredibly heavy weight that causes you to fail at 3 reps. So, in this instance, instead of moving the weight as fast as you can, you lower it in a controlled movement and explode up on the positive or concentric part of the movement. For example, if you're doing a barbell bench press, to build muscular power traditionally, you move the weight as quickly and explosively as possible for 1-5 reps. This will build muscular power but will do little for changing the shape and size of the muscle. However, if you increase the repetitions to eight or even ten, slow down the eccentric (negative or lowering) part of the rep and explode on the concentric (positive) part of the rep. This will give you the best of both worlds. More muscular power and an increase in fibre tears can lead to more muscle growth, size and power. To really understand this concept and allow you to change your body composition, while making yourself stronger, fitter and faster, it helps to understand how muscle actions actually work.

Muscle Actions:

Concentric Muscle Actions:

These occur when a muscle shortens during contraction. An example of a concentric muscle action is the upward phase of a bench press, as mentioned above.

Eccentric Muscle Actions:

These are the reverse of concentric actions. The muscle returns to its original starting point The muscle lengthens as the joint angle increases, releasing under controlled tension. Examples of eccentric actions include the lowering of the bench press. The repetition tempo (the speed or count of a lift, time under load tension) you use with concentric and eccentric actions will determine how the muscle responds. For example, the more time the muscle is under tension in the eccentric portion of a movement, the more fibres you will tear. Combining slow eccentric actions with fast concentric ones is a great way to build explosive power.

Isometric Muscle Actions:

These occur when the muscle develops tension without changing its length. For example, an isometric contraction develops during a bicep curl if you cannot continue the movement beyond the midpoint. The same thing happens when you hold a bodyweight front or side plank.

Prime Move/Agonist:

The muscle that brings about a movement is called the prime mover or agonist. For example, during a bicep curl, the prime mover is the bicep muscle.

Antagonist:

The muscle that acts in opposition to the prime mover, which may slow it down or stop the movement, is called the antagonist. It helps to keep the joint stable and it is released during most movements, allowing the movement to be performed efficiently. For example, during a bicep curl, the triceps (the three muscles on the back of your arm, 'tri' meaning three) act as the antagonist and need to be relaxed in order to allow the arm to be flexed smoothly.

Although eccentric, concentric and isometric are the three most important muscle actions to understand for this program as well as in general, if you're an advanced trainer (following programs for five years or more), it can also help to understand how agonist and antagonist muscle actions work when trying to fully engage a muscle during any particular movement or exercise in your program.

Muscle structure, muscle fibre types and mind-muscle connection

Muscles make up about 45% of an average person's body weight. They are 80% water, and the rest is mostly protein. Each muscle is made up of cylindrical fibres, often referred to as muscle cells or muscle fibres. You cannot change the number of fibres in your muscle, but you can increase both the cross sectional area, through strength and resistance training, and the number of muscle fibres recruited when executing any given movement. Your muscle fibre types can be classified into two types.

- Slow-twitch (ST) or type 1 fibres
- Fast-twitch (FT) or type 2 fibres

Slow-twitch fibres

Slow-twitch fibres are used for endurance activities, long-distance running for example. They contract relatively slowly, produce less tension and prefer to use oxygen to produce energy (i.e. aerobic metabolism). Slow-twitch fibres can easily make use of both fat and carbohydrate for fuel. One of the reason that people do low-intensity, steady-state (LISS) cardio, i.e. jog or brisk walk, normally comes down to the ease at which the body can use fat as a fuel source when all other things, such as macro timings, calorie intake and overall nutrition, are considered. You will see in the nutrition section of the book that fast-twitch muscle fibres use carbohydrates much more effectively; hence, it is so crucial for sprint-sport athletes. Slow-twitch fibres do not tire easily so are used for nearly all low-intensity, long-duration aerobic activities such as walking and jogging.

I remember from the age of nineteen to twenty-two, every season when we started training again, the longer runs used to make me feel sick for the first two months. My muscular system was never able to sustain it and, every January and February, I would beat myself up for 'becoming unfit' in the off season. This, however, wasn't actually true. I was always in the weight room or the gym lifting or using resistance training to build myself up over the winter months, but it never helped me for that first month of training. Over the past several years, I've been very fortunate to work with so many athletes as their strength and conditioning coach through my programs and, year after year, I observed this same pattern occurring with them as well.

After three or four off-season cycles, I realsed that I was losing nearly two months of training every year as I tried to regain my aerobic fitness. These were two months that I could have focused on improving my strength further, improving my glute activation so as to be faster to the ball or working on the weaker areas of my game to provide me with a psychological edge in games.

A lot of the athletes who come through my programs had the exact same problem. This is one of the reasons I add aerobic 'slow-twitch focus' activity to the off-season programs (2-5 km aerobic zone runs 2-4 times a week depending on each person's goals, position, level, etc.). When you think about all the other higher-priority areas that you could improve upon at the start of a new season, the physical and psychological edge that it can give you over everybody else can have a significant impact on your performance over the course of an entire season. This, alongside certain personality traits, is probably one of the reasons that my athletes tend to excel to the top of their club teams or break into (and in some cases, dominate) their county times. They say you should work smarter and not harder, but if you work smart and hard, you really become a force to be reckoned with.

Fast-twitch fibres

Fast-twitch fibres are essentially the opposite of slow-twitch fibres. They are best suited to anaerobic activities – anything requiring more than 25% of your maximum strength. These fibres can generate high levels of tension, contract very rapidly but have poor endurance. Fast-twitch fibres can be further subdivided into fast-twitch type IIa and fast-twitch type IIb. This is based on their ability to produce energy under aerobic conditions. Fast-twitch type IIa fibres are more resistant to fatigue, while fast-twitch type IIb fibres tire quickly and are used almost exclusively for explosive power, sprinting, jumping, etc.

Each muscle has a combination of fast-twitch and slow-twitch fibres. This is largely genetically determined, in the sense that you are genetically more inclined to have more of one or the other. For example, a sprinter is more likely to have more fast-twitch muscle fibres while a marathon runner will more likely have more slow-twitch muscle fibres.

Many believe that there is not much you can do about your genetics, but modern science and the field of epigenetics in particular are starting to publish studies on how we can alter our genetics through diet and lifestyle changes. Even though you are more inclined to lean towards your own genetic type, it doesn't mean you can't have the best of both worlds.

Personally, I spent most of my life as a fast-twitch athlete – GAA, soccer, Crossfit and bodybuilding, to name a few undertakings – but I've also completed marathons, triathlons and ultra-marathons. The philosophy in this book comes down to taking the very best from all disciplines and merging them into a system that allows your performance and physique to reach its maximum potential. Bodybuilding is incredible at changing the composition and shape of the muscle, Crossfit is great at working high-volume metabolic conditioning (especially in controlled parameters) and running, albeit for notably shorter distances than say a marathon (3-5 km), is great for building your aerobic endurance and improving the recruitment of slow-twitch muscle fibres. When you combine the best of all disciplines and all worlds, you get the best of all disciplines and all worlds.

Mind-muscle connection

Have you ever just moved a weight from A to B, not really feeling any particular muscle? You know it hurts and you are clearly working out, but you can't really pinpoint what muscle you worked? This happens due to a lack of a mind-muscle connection.

It's exactly as it sounds. You want your mind connected to the muscle you are working. For example, if you are doing a dumbbell bent over row, you want to feel your back during each rep. However, the closest muscles to your grip are your forearms and bicep. Therefore, normally those muscles can kick in and fatigue before you have even worked your back. This is where your training systems really shines, because you are not moving weight from A to B; you are moving a weight with perfect form, creating optimal tension or explosiveness on the muscle you are trying to work (back in this case) from A to B. This way, you can create more tension or explosiveness in the muscle without having to go 'very heavy', effectively reducing your risk of injury.

For example, in my current training program, I can only lift 4 or 5 kg during side lateral raises for the shoulders. If you are able to lift 25 kg during this movement, you either have super human strength or you are swinging with momentum, meaning that you are not working the muscle for optimal tension. The best piece of gym advice that I have received was, 'Leave your ego at the door.' I generally find women much better at this, but here's an added note for any men reading this – if you are trying to achieve a leaner, toned and more muscular physique, but feel the need to constantly out-lift your training partners with super heavy weight during a bench press or a barbell curl, it might be worth considering changing your training partners.

Don't get me wrong, you still want to find a weight that is heavy enough to allow you to fail at your given rep range and tempo. When I say I use 5 kg for side lateral raises, that's the heaviest weight I can physically lift with perfect form, creating optimal tension on the side deltoid – the muscle I'm working. You may need to use 10 kg or 12 kg to create the same tension. Just be careful not to swing the weight with momentum. With the exception of a system called 'cheat reps', where you use a slight momentum at the end of an exercise when you hit muscular failure, if you are doing it from your first rep, it's just bad form.

Building a mind-muscle connection with every body part doesn't happen overnight, and you will find it much harder to connect with certain exercises or body parts than with others. For example, it took me years to learn to 'feel' my legs when I trained them. I would move a weight from A to B, and my legs never really responded. It wasn't until I learnt about creating optimal muscular tension and started implementing it in my own training that they responded. Now, they are probably my strongest body parts. So, if you struggle to feel your glutes, chest or biceps, remember that I was there too. However, with the right system, you can turn your weakest body part into your strongest.

Form: it's not about the weight, it's about how you move the weight

Creating optimal tension, working for explosiveness and feeling the muscle you are trying to work is indeed the secret to better body composition and performance. However, you also need to do it right. When you hear people talking about their 'form', it's actually just the way they do a certain movement. If you do a barbell bent over row with a curved back, that's considered 'bad form', which basically means that you're not performing the movement in the correct way. As mentioned above, I'm not asking you to go super light. You want to pick a weight that enables you to perform the movements within the perfect form and fail at the given rep range.

How muscles work

Your muscles are connected to your nervous system. They are fired, or activated, by motor nerves, and a single motor nerve may stimulate anywhere between one and several hundred muscle fibres. One of the reasons that compound lifts (squat, bench, military press, pull-ups, etc.) work so effectively for athletes is because of the increased amount of muscles that are stimulated in those movements. For example, if you do a bicep curl, you're largely only recruiting your bicep muscles (two small muscles at the front of your arm). However, when you are doing a barbell squat, not only are you recruiting your quads, hamstrings and glutes, but your entire core has to brace and strengthen itself in order to stabilise the weight during each repetition. These are what I call 'better bang for your buck' exercises – you get more benefit in less time. It's based off the scientific 'size principle' – as training load increases, progressively more muscle fibres are activated or engaged. Three sets of barbell squats are going to recruit more muscle fibres than ten sets of bicep curls. That being said, I regularly factor biceps movements into my program too. I just advise not doing them at the beginning of workouts when you are at your freshest; start with your hardest, biggest or 'most muscle recruited' exercise first and then move to smaller body parts during the workout as you start to get tired and fatigued.

Light vs. heavy weight

A nerve cell and a muscle fibre together are called a motor unit. When a motor nerve is stimulated, it causes all the muscle fibres to contract. This is normally called the 'all or nothing principle' i.e. a muscle fibre either contracts or it doesn't and when it does, it contracts with maximum force. The number of motor units involved in a contraction depends on the load imposed on the muscle. When you use 'light' weights, less muscles fibres are recruited. As the load increases, progressively more motor units will be recruited, activating the fast-twitch fibres – until, with a maximum weight, most of the motor units are recruited.

Note: The meaning of 'light' is subjective. When I say light, I mean that if you were aiming for 8 repetitions of an exercise with a 10 kg weight and could have done 15 or 16 repetitions, the weight was 'too light'. This is why it's so important to pick the right weight to fail at your given rep range and track it every week so that you're not losing out on potential strength or muscle gains. To stimulate the whole muscle, you have to work with weights that require all-out effort, regardless of the parameters you are working within. This is the same for a bicep curl, where you are only really engaging one or two muscles, compared to a squat, where you are engaging several muscles together. The only difference is the number of muscles that are actually being recruited. The principle remains the same.

How to pick the right weight

For example, if you're doing a barbell squat, working for a tempo of 4:1:2 (four seconds lowering, one second pause at the bottom and two seconds on the way back up) and you have picked a weight that you can easily complete 9, 10 or 11 reps with, that particular weight is too light and you need to go heavier.

Conversely, if you're aiming for 8 reps and fail at 5 or 6 reps, the weight is too heavy and you need to reduce it. The key is to keep track of the weight you used and always try to fail at your given rep range.

How muscles grow

Increase in strength is the combined result of changes in the way nerve pathways serve the motor units – neuromuscular adaptions – and developing bigger muscles – hypertrophy.

Hypertrophy is when you use your training to force your muscles to do more work than normal to overcome the load. This process is called overloading and leads to an increase in muscle strength and size through a process called hypertrophy. When you hear the term 'bodybuilding', 'hypertrophy' or even 'hypertrophy parameters', they normally all refer to the same thing – overloading a muscle in a given rep, rest and set range. Hypertrophy parameters are normally 8-10 reps, with 45-60 seconds rest with 3-4 sets.

Thus, neuromuscular adaption can be described as the changes in the way the nerve pathways serve the motor unit. It's a type of motor learning – your body learns to assign more and more motor units to the movements to make you stronger. When you begin lifting weights, most of the strength gains come from the nerves controlling the muscle-firing pattern, and they learn how to become more efficient over time. The nervous system adapts to a progressive overload by improving its ability to recruit additional muscle fibres in order to generate more force.

At twelve years old, I remember the first time I ever tried to move a 20 kg barbell on a bench. The bar seemed to push up my right side (my dominant side), slowly followed by my left, in what can only be described as a zig-zag motion; I felt like I was pushing against the world. After what felt like 20 minutes (it was actually about 6 seconds), I got the bar up into a locked position. This 'struggle', where you feel like the bar or weight is shifting from one side to the other, is your nervous system creating that new 'neural pathway'.

The analogy I like is that of going through a jungle. The first time you go through, you have to chop small trees, push through bushes, basically forge a brand new path. But every time you take that same path, it becomes progressively clearer and easier to follow. The same mechanism occurs with lifting weights and your nervous system. The first time you try and 'go through the jungle', i.e. move the weight in a new movement pattern, it's hard because your body has never performed that movement under that load. I experience the same thing every time I try to learn a new skill, exercise or technique for something. The more you perform the movement pattern, the stronger the neural pathways become and the easier the activity becomes.

This same principle applies when you are trying to learn a new skill that's transferrable to the pitch. I made my senior debut for my club when I was fifteen and at the time, I was predominantly left-footed. That was the season during which the weak points of my game were really exposed for the first time. I was playing against fully-grown men and, although I was fast and relatively strong for my age, it wasn't enough at that level. The smart corner-backs realised pretty quickly that I could only kick with my left foot and simply pushed me onto my weaker side so I couldn't shoot. Soon, I realised that I was going to have to learn how to kick with my weaker foot if I was going to make any impact that season.

I remember practising for the first time in my backyard at home, and it felt like somebody else was taking control of my body. I was dropping the ball with my left hand onto my right foot, which made me look like a tangled octopus – it felt so incredibly awkward. As funny as that picture may be, this is normally the first mistake that occurs when learning to kick or puck with your weaker side. Your nervous system is so hardwired to dropping the ball with your left hand onto your left foot, or right hand onto your right foot, that it's like trying to write new computer code from scratch.

I practised every day for about two months, and it got better and progressively stronger with every week. The new pathways were forming. Now, in my thirties, even though I only play recreationally due to my endurance events, I can still kick equally well with both feet and have done so since I was eighteen. **Practice doesn't make perfect, practice makes permanent**. Understanding the neural pathways and that the process is exactly the same whether learning to kick or puck with your weaker side, learning a new movement in thy gym or learning a new instrument for the first time. The concept will always remain exactly the same.

After this initial neural pathway period, as you increase the load (the weight you're lifting) during exercises, you muscles start to grow in size, which can massively contribute to strength gains as well. Strength and size aren't the same thing, nor are they completely different. You can get stronger and not add any size, or you can add size without getting stronger.

For example, when I used to compete as a competitive bodybuilder, I would regularly add size or mass to body parts such as my shoulders, but the actually 'weight' I lifted would never increase. I would change the angles and vary the rep ranges, but my dumbbell shoulder press never really went above 30 kg for 6-8 reps. That being said, in the majority of cases, you are going to get both – if you focus on building size, your strength will increase, and if you focus on building strength, you will see an increase in size. The key for achieving both is working with the correct load, i.e. choosing the right weight using the directions mentioned above, and focusing on performing all movements with perfect form to recruit all the fibres you are trying to focus on, thereafter recovering effectively after each workout.

You don't build muscle in the gym

The repeated contraction of muscles during resistance training damages the muscle tissue. The muscle proteins (actin and myosin) undergo micro-trauma, and microscopic tears occur in the muscle fibres and connective tissue. This occurs primarily during the eccentric (negative) phase of an exercise and normally causes the soreness you feel for a few days after an intense workout. You don't grow or get stronger in the gym, you tear down muscle fibres and actually make yourself 'weaker' in the gym – it's your food, recovery and sleep after you train that allows you to increase size and improve strength. Remember, training is a stressor, albeit a positive and controlled one. However, your body has a basic survival mechanism, and the stress that you undergo during hard physical training sends the message to your body that you need to get 'stronger' or 'bigger' to deal with this workload again in the future. During rest periods between workouts, new proteins are built up, the connective tissue is repaired, muscle fibres enlarge and the muscle increases in size and strength. This is why a good recovery strategy that focuses on your nutrition and sleep is so crucial.

Developing speed, agility and reflexes

For all athletes, the ability to quickly change direction often decides the difference between success and failure. GAA involves whole body movements that require you to rapidly and instantly accelerate, decelerate (slow down) or change direction in response to game situations. For example, it's very common for a corner-forward to make a short run, double back and then attempt a zig-zag movement to other side to retrieve the ball. If you're marking the forward, you have to mimic the same movement patterns to try and stay in front of him. In GAA, the ability to charge direction is just as important as great straight-line sprinting. Agility can be broken down into subcomponents made up of both physical qualities and cognitive abilities. The focus of the next section is to example the physical qualities of speed and agility along with the importance of glute activation to maximise 'take-off' speed and improve your sprinting capabilities.

Speed

The old adage 'speed kills' is probably as true for sports as for anything else. Athletes who can move faster than their opponents have the advantage. For example, a fast corner-back can get to the ball more quickly than the forward he's marking or the centre-forward can outrun a centre-back when receiving a pass from midfield. Speed is often measured by using linear (straight line) sprinting over a distance between 40 and 100 metres. However, it's worth noting that, as important as straight line sprinting is, most athletes in GAA rarely sprint more than 30 metres in a straight line before they make some type of directional change. Thus, it's always worth having some multidimensional or unilateral (one side a time) movements as a part of your training regimen.

Stabilisation and speed

Joint stability is an important and often overlooked

factor that contributes to the effective application of force during sprinting and take-off. Agility training requires strengthening of the muscles involved in stabilising the trunk and the joints of your lower body. Not only can this make you physically stronger on the ball, so that you can give and receive tackles more effectively, but can also improve your overall speed, as your muscles activate more rapidly. Resistance training exercises can enhance the strength and activation of the muscles you require for stabilisation. Both bilateral (both sides) and unilateral (one side) drills, such as the ones listed below, work extremely well.

- Multi-joint or compound movements such as the back or front squat and forward, reverse and diagonal lunges
- Single-limb training such as single-leg squats (leaning back on a TRX or band for example)
- Explosive plyometric movements performed with correct form, such as box jumps or clapping push-ups

Intramuscular coordination is another important aspect of muscular contractions that is closely related to stability during movement. Each muscle can send signals and information to the other muscles in the system. The ease and speed at which they communicate relates to the activation timing of the various muscles across the joints. In simpler terms, the more often the muscles are used to 'firing' or 'switching on', the quicker and faster they will activate.

Intramuscular coordination is important for running speed, because if the hamstrings are not relaxed when the thigh is brought forward in the recovery phase of the stride, hip flexion will be reduced, resulting in a shorter stride length. This is especially clear in movements involving directional changes, where joint stability is of greater concern for the athlete. One of my favourite athletes, Cristiano Ronaldo, is arguably the best athlete in the world at doing this. His ability to change direction at speed is incredible to witness. When you think 'intramuscular coordination' or using resistance training to improve your ability to change direction at speed, think about Ronaldo when he was twenty-seven or twenty-eight years old.

The key to maximise this is to build the right amount of multi-joint/compound movements, single leg and plyometric training, along with the proper recovery strategy to keep hip flexors and hamstrings loose with maximum glute activation on every multidimensional and straight-line sprint.

Your brain and speed!

The ability to identify relevant cues and execute the correct corresponding movements without delay largely determines any player's success. If a player misreads or mistimes these cues, it can literally cost possession, a goal or even a game. Numerous decision-making factors influence your reactive ability, or quickness, which can have a huge impact on your game. When your brain is working clearly, you can make better and faster decisions, which can give you a huge edge over any opponent. The nutrition section of the book has more information about how to use certain foods to potentially reduce the inflammation in your body as well as talks about supplements that can stimulate your sympathetic nervous system to enable your brain to work optimally on rest, training and, most importantly, game days.

Information processing

According to R.A Schmidte and Wrisberg C.A, in their book *Human Kinetics*, before athletes move, they must first identify the need to respond to a situation. They do this by collecting environmental cues from a variety of sensory input systems, such as auditory, visual and somatosensory systems.

Note: The somatosensory system is the part of the sensory system concerned with the conscious perception of touch, pressure, pain, temperature, position, movement and vibration, which arise from the muscles, joints, skin and fascia.

For example, a midfielder waits for the goalkeeper to provide the auditory command to signal the start of play on a kick or puck out, i.e. he shouts that it's coming in that direction. As he prepares to jump for the kick or puck out, he collects visual information about the position of his marker in an attempt to time his jump. As other players try and tackle him, he reaches up for the ball, his somatosensory system gives his central nervous system feedback about the manual pressure the opponents are applying to him as he jumps. Using this information, the player may be able to cut away from the attack. This scenario illustrates just one situation where environmental cues provide athletes with important information about their competitive environment during play. The reason I have shared this is that certain supplements that stimulate the sympathetic nervous system, such as caffeine, can heighten awareness in these situations and improve your overall reaction time. This is discussed in more detail in the supplements section of the book.

Decision-making skills

Once you have collected information about the environment and the situation (e.g. should you run for the next ball or double back, zig-zag and then look for it on the next play?), you must decide which actions or responses will yield the greatest success. Successful decision-making requires both speed and precise movement. When you have decided which specific movement to make based on the information collected from the environment, a message is sent to your motor cortex to retrieve the desired movement pattern from your memory. Whatever drill it is you are practising, always focus on proper technique. My favourite example of this is taken from another sport. Former professional NBA player Larry Bird, who was known for becoming one of the top names in the sports history owing to his sheer work ethic over his natural genetic ability, reportedly used to practice free throws with a blindfold on. This forced his body to repeat the same shooting form and also helped him visualise his shots better. I'm not necessarily saying you should blindfold yourself when practicing shots; I am asking you to practice the drills that you need to improve. Resistance training, your nutritional plan and your recovery strategy will put you at the peak of your physical performance, but that alone won't improve your passing or get the ball over the bar in games. Putting it all together is what separates the good from the great.

Anticipation

If you can accurately predict an event or plan movements in advance, you can initiate an appropriate response more quickly than if you had waited to react to a given stimulus. For example, if you're marking a forward that can only kick or puck from one side, you can put pressure on this side, forcing him to make a mistake. With experience, you can gain greater knowledge of how long it takes to coordinate your own movements relative to certain environmental regularities and opponent tendencies in a given situation. In addition, if you can predict which play will be used and when it will occur, you will be able to form an appropriate response before the stimulus is presented. For example, if you know that your goalkeeper touches his head before he kicks or pucks out to the right-hand side, you know in advance whether to make a run or not. In nearly all cases, this can be trained by wiring your central nervous system to execute certain movements patterns and then conditioning your muscle memory so that you can react faster than your opponents. I remember when I suffered my last knee injury at the age of twenty-one (my third knee dislocation). I was unable to kick with my left foot when I first came back (I had injured my right side and it wasn't strong enough for me to balance my body). My club mate Declan Kyne, who I grew up with, (he has played in the full-back line for Galway footballers for the last three years as of writing this) would always mark me during training. Growing up, he was generally always at full- or centre-back, and I was full- or centre-forward on our club team. I remember the frustration I felt for being able to turn only to one side. Declan knew I couldn't use my left foot with my injury and just keep pushing me onto that side. I don't think I scored at a single training session for an entire month! Athletes who possess the ability to anticipate accurately can gain a large competitive advantage over their opposition, as demonstrated by Declan's example.

How do I get abs?

Becoming an amazing athlete that's fitter, faster and stronger with a leaner and more muscular physique basically depends on the combination of your nutrition, your training, your recovery and your direct-skill work on the pitch. However, there's one last piece to the training puzzle that nearly every athlete desires (well, I did anyways), and that's getting abs or a six pack.

There's a reason why so many athletes have trouble seeing their abs, and it has nothing to do with the amount of cardio they do. Most athletes train on the pitch at least twice a week with a game on the weekend. Schools, college, underage and inter-county players train even more than that, so if it was only about cardio, nearly every athlete would have a six pack.

Instead, it's that most players are misinformed about what it takes to make their abs show. It's the combination of your nutrition (getting your body fat low enough to see abs), the right core movements (compound lifts with concentric and isosmotic ab moves) and your cardio on the pitch that you are required to get right in order for you to carve out your midsection. When I went on my second J1 student working visa in California, after five or six nights a week of frat parties, bars and clubs, I had put on some very unwanted bodyfat and was pushing the scales at a not-very-defined 86 kg. Up until that point, I had been lifting in the gym and playing with a senior club in San Francisco, but my abs were nowhere to be seen. I grew up on a farm with a meat and potatoes diet, so staying big and strong was never too difficult, but maintaining that size and having abs at the same time was always a lot harder. That was the first time in my life I was truly 'out of shape' – I saw photos of myself from a trip to Las Vegas (that I regrettably destroyed at the time due to embarrassment) and decided that I had to get myself back on track ASAP. I went back to a clean eating plan, reduced my alcohol intake (reduced, not eliminated, I was a student after all), cut out the fast food I was eating and set out on the path of getting abs again.

My ab training focused on activating the muscles in the abdomen at full capacity with a mixture of compound lifts, concentric and isometric movements and, most importantly, burning away all the layers of fat that were covering the deep cuts of the muscles. A lot of my knowledge on how to go from 20+% body fat to having visible abs at 13% and lower came from this period in my life. It took me about a year to put all the pieces together, but if you learn from my mistakes, it will take you significantly less time.

At the end of the day, you can have the strongest abs in the world, but if you have too much fat on your stomach, you won't see them. Power lifters are a great example of this. At first glance, most look muscular and kind of fat. From a strength standpoint, they have insanely strong, powerful and dense abs for holding, moving and lifting heavy weight. The big difference is that their diets aren't designed to reduce fat and their training isn't designed to make them leaner. The opposite can be said for somebody who has a skinny, ectomorph body type. They may have abs but usually have a really weak core. It's normally pretty easy to tell if someone's core is weak, they can't hold a plank for any noteworthy length of time and can't stabilise their core during barbell or front squats. In most cases of ectomorph body types, they have the opposite problem; they have abs and they're lean but they want to add more weight, muscle or size to their frame. See 'Create your own weight gainer shake' in the nutrition section for more information on this.

So, you can have a strong core but not a six pack or you can have a six pack but not a strong core. The intention in this book is to get you both! Having a strong core is vital for breaking through tackles and improving your overall performance, while abs are the icing on the cake for most physiques. If you're wondering how to build a bigger, leaner and faster physique with a six pack to go with it, read on.

Ab training 101 for athletes

Your abs are an extremely complex muscle group. They are made up of a combination of several layers, cross sections and muscles. Bruce lee was famous for doing a thousand sit ups per night. It was his performance in martial arts that gave birth to the perception that doing an insane number of daily abs exercises was the only way to go. While Bruce Lee did have an incredible core, you don't need to do what he did to get a six pack. In the case of getting abs, it's all about quality over quantity. I have my athletes work their abs two to three times per week, usually with a bodyweight movement, an isometric hold or a Swiss ball movement; however, the focus is on hitting them efficiently. For years, I used to do abs at the end of my workout but now, I think it's better to mix it up on different days. For example, you can have a Swiss ball plank at the start of your workout on Monday, a hanging leg raise in the middle of your workout on Wednesday and bodyweight ab crossovers at the end of your workout on Friday. The key is to recruit your abs in nearly all of your workouts – as long as you have a mixture of compound lifts with direct abs movements, you are going to create enough muscular stimulation to start seeing them shape up and strengthen as your body fat lowers. After that, it's just about getting your body fat low enough through proper nutrition.

Sample training program

Similar to the nutrition sample earlier, this is an extremely basic tester workout that you can try. Of course, it's always best to have a training program based around your specific goals, your current schedule and to make sure that it's working around your lifestyle. However, here is a sample workout that you can try, which incorporates the best of hypertrophy, strength work and metabolic conditioning. The amount of gym sessions in any program will vary depending on whether it's off, pre- or mid-season; but, for this one, try adding it in once or twice a week along with your current training or instead of your current gym program.

Training program details

Exercise:

The name of the exercise you will perform.

Sets:

The number of sets is the number of 'rounds' you do. For example, if you do 3 sets of 10 reps, you perform 10 reps of the exercise with a 2:1:2 tempo and then rest for

60 seconds. Repeat for your second and third set.

<u>Reps:</u>

Reps are the number of repetitions you will do, i.e. the number of times you will perform the movements; for example, if you do the movement 10 times, that's 10 reps. The aim is to work till 'failure' – doing as many reps as you physically can till you can't do any more or physically fail.

<u>Rest:</u> The amount of time you rest in between sets.

<u>Tempo:</u>

This is the speed at which you perform the exercise. For example, 2:1:2 means that you spend two seconds on the positive (the upward or downward motion), 1 second on the squeeze (at the top or bottom depending on the exercise) and 2 seconds on the negative (the downward or upward motion). It's worth noting that if you have never worked under a strict tempo, you will more than likely be using less weight than you normally would for certain exercises. This is normally just for a week or two until your muscles strengthen and adjust to the new tempo.

<u>Superset:</u>

This is when you perform the first move followed by the next move without any rest in between. For example, doing 10 repetitions of box jumps followed by 10 repetitions of plyometric push-ups, then rest.

Timing for each workout:

This workout should take about 45 minutes. It is about quality over quantity; therefore, carry a stopwatch to time your rest periods, train intensely while in the gym and get out within 45 minutes so that you don't begin to burn through any hard-earned muscle or overstress your central nervous system.

Track your weight:

As the weeks progress, your body will get stronger in each exercise; therefore, increase the weight every week (if required) so that you fail in the given rep range for each workout.

For example, if you're lifting 20 kg during barbell back squats, you may need to increase this to 22.5 kg after one or two weeks as your muscles get stronger.

You can do this workout once, twice or even three times per week. For information on more workouts, check out my social media channels 'Brian Keane' and 'Brian Keane Fitness' or to look into my GAA Lean Body Program, go to www.briankeanefitness.com

Exercise 1: Barbell back squats

Sets: 3

Reps: 8-10

Rest: 90 seconds

Tempo: 4:1:1 (four seconds lowering, one second pause at the bottom, explode up)

Description:

1. Stand with your feet slightly wider than your shoulders. Most people prefer to turn their toes out to 30 degrees, but this is personal preference.

2. Place the barbell across your upper back. You can place the bar above or below your shoulder blades. Just ensure that it is comfortably in place and doesn't move around during the reps.

3. Take a deep breath, and descend into the squat.

4. Squat down until your thighs are parallel with the ground, pushing your knees out over your toes.

5. Rise upwards, making sure to squeeze your quads (or glutes depending on your focus) to lockout.

Exercise 2: Box jump superset with spider push-ups

Sets: 3

Reps: 10 reps of box jumps and 8 reps each side for spider push-ups

Rest: 90 seconds

Tempo: 2:1:2

Description:

Box jump:

1. Begin with placing a box of an appropriate height (one you can comfortably jump and land on) 1-2 feet in front of you. Stand with your feet shoulder width apart. This will be your starting position.

2. Perform a short squat in preparation for jumping, swinging your arms behind you.

3. Rebound out of this position, extending through the hips, knees and ankles to jump as high as possible. Swing your arms forward and up.

4. Land on the box with the knees bent, absorbing the impact through the legs. You can jump from the box back to the ground or preferably step down one leg at a time.

Spider Push-Up:

1. Begin in a push-up position on the floor. Support your weight on your hands and toes, with your feet together and your body straight in a full-push or press-up position. Your arms should be bent at 90 degrees. This will be your starting position.

2. Initiate the movement by raising one foot off the ground. Rotate the leg externally and bring the knee toward your elbow as far forward as possible as you drop into a push-up.

3. Return this leg to the starting position and repeat on the opposite side. Perform 8 reps on both sides for a total of 16 reps.

Variations:

•   If you are new to this exercise and do not have the strength to perform it, perform the movement as is without the push-up element. Now, you bring your knees to your elbows in a slow and controlled manner without a push- or press-up in between each repetition.

Exercise 3: Pull-ups

Sets: 3

Reps: Failure

Rest: 60 seconds

Tempo: 2:1:2

Description:

1. Grab the pull-up bar with the palms facing forward and a shoulder-width grip.

2. While you have both arms extended in front of you holding the bar, bring your torso back by around 30 degrees or so while curving your lower back and sticking your chest out. This is your starting position.

3. Pull your torso up until the bar touches your upper chest by drawing the shoulders and the upper arms down and back. Exhale as you perform this portion of the movement. **Tip:** Concentrate on squeezing the back muscles once you reach the fully contracted position. The upper torso should remain stationary as it moves through space and only the arms should move. The forearms should not do any other work besides hold the bar.

4. After a second in the contracted position, start to inhale and slowly lower your torso back to the starting

position, where your arms are fully extended and the lats are fully stretched.

5. Repeat this motion for as many repetitions as possible until you fail. Aim for a minimum of 5 and a maximum of 20 repetitions.

Variations:

- If you are new to this exercise and do not have the strength to perform it, use a chin assist machine if available. These machines use weights to help push your bodyweight.

- If a chin assist machine is not available, a spotter holding your legs can help, or you can use a band to help you with the movement.

Exercise 4: Dumbbell alternating rear lunge superset Swiss ball plank

Sets: 3

Reps: 10 reps on each side for reverse lunges and 30-60 seconds of swiss ball plank

Rest: 90 seconds

Tempo: 2:1:2 and isometric static hold

Description:

Dumbbell Alternating Rear Lunge

1. Stand with your torso upright holding two dumbbells in your hands by your sides. This will be your starting position.

2. Step backward with your right leg around two feet or so with your left foot and lower your upper body while keeping the torso upright and maintaining balance. Inhale as you go down. **Tip:** As in the other exercises, do not allow your knee to go forward beyond your toes as you come down, as this will put undue stress on the knee joint. Make sure that you keep the shin of your front leg perpendicular to the ground. Keep the torso upright during the lunge; flexible hip flexors are important. A long lunge emphasises the gluteus maximus (glutes), while a short lunge emphasises quadriceps.

3. Push up and go back to the starting position as you exhale. **Tip:** Use the balls of your feet to push in order to accentuate the quadriceps. To focus on the glutes, press with your heels.

4. Now repeat this with the opposite leg.

Variations:

- You can perform this as a bodyweight only movement as well.

- Another alternative is to perform all your repetitions with one leg before alternating to the other leg. Experiment with both and figure out what works best for you.

Swiss Ball Plank:

1. Get into a prone position on the Swiss ball, supporting your weight on your toes and your forearms on the Swiss ball. Your arms are bent directly below the shoulder.

2. Keep your body straight at all times and hold this position for 30-60 seconds.

Variations:

To decrease difficulty, remove the Swiss ball and perform the same movement on the floor like a normal plank.

CHAPTER 4:

SLEEP

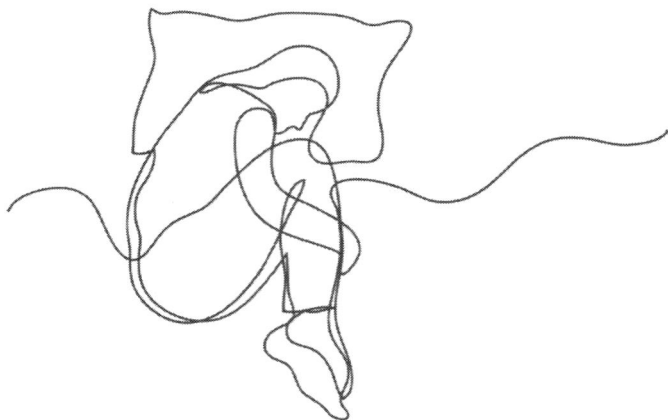

Sleep for Athletes

Finally, we get to the ultimate piece of the puzzle as well as the last foundation pillar for getting into incredible shape and raising your physique and performance to the next level. If training and nutrition (along with supplements) are the first two foundation pillars, then sleep is definitely the third.

As someone who has been a notoriously poor sleeper most of his life, it's very simple for me to see how easily poor sleep quality can not only affect your physical performance on the pitch but also your overall life quality in general. Poor sleep can influence everything from your energy levels during training sessions to your willpower and ability to make better food choices throughout the day.

See if this situation is familiar in anyway. You wake up to the alarm on your phone and reach over to turn it off. While you're there, you check the notifications you received overnight from social media, emails and texts from work and friends. Your mouth is dry, your brain feels like it's still somewhat asleep, there's light leaking in through the curtain and you can see the stand-by light of the TV, laptop or whichever other device you were using at the foot of the bed, staring unblinking at you, reminding you of what you were watching right before you feel asleep last night. This was my morning routine for the better part of my twenties, and if you're like a lot of my athletes, yours won't differ too much. If that was you this morning, I just want you to ask yourself one question – did you sleep well?

According to Nick Littlehales, in his great book *Sleep*, the average person in Britain and Ireland gets a little over six and half hours of sleep a night. It's a pretty similar story all around the western world – people in the US get slightly less, people in Canada get slightly more and so on. However, there is an exception to this general-population rule – professional athletes. These individuals know that recovery and performance benefits are highly correlated with improved sleep quality and have been taking advantage of it for at least the past decade. My hope is to show you that you don't have to be a professional athlete to take full advantage of improving your overall sleep quality and how implementing a few night-time routines and sleep hacks can improve your mental cognition (your ability to react faster on the pitch), your physical recovery (your ability to recover muscularly between sessions, workouts and games) and improve your overall energy levels throughout the day so you don't fatigue and fail at crucial times during games or training sessions.

The problem with poor sleep

In *The Fitness Mindset*, I spoke about how we waste time falling asleep and spend hours in a light sleep state as well as how that doesn't give us the same body- and brain-boosting benefits of deep REM (rapid eye movement) sleep.

Personally, in the past, I would spend an hour trying to fall asleep because my brain wouldn't stop rehashing the day's events; this was especially true when I was a player, as every mistake I made in games or during training would replay over and over in my head at night. Now, don't get me wrong, this kind of self-evaluation on performance can be a very positive thing; it tells you exactly where your game needs to improve and gives you direct feedback on what you have to work on. If you were getting pushed off the ball, you may need to start doing more bodyweight or gym work to get stronger. If you missed two of your five shots at goal, you need to practise your shooting, or if you were beaten constantly to every fifty-fifty ball, you may need to start working on your acceleration to quicken your take-off. This self-analysis is important and the best players I work with do it regularly. But when you're trying to wind down and fall asleep, it isn't the best time to think about it. If you're the kind of person who overthinks your performance and replays mistakes over and over again in your head, my advice is to designate a time specifically for doing this – either by yourself or with a friend, partner or coach. Go over exactly what you did well and what you need to improve upon. Write it down somewhere, even if you never look at it again. There's certain mental catharsis we can get from writing down things that we need to work on and then, we can leave it or come back to it in the future. I guarantee if it's playing over and over in your head, writing it down will make you feel a lot better and help you reduce your overthinking or anxiety after games or training sessions. I learnt this technique from former Irish rugby captain Paul O'Connell and have used it very successfully with some of my athletes ever since.

During my mid-twenties, I actually started perceiving sleep as a waste of time. I tried different supplements, going to bed earlier, going to bed later, but I would still wake up groggy every morning and never really feel like I had fully recovered. I'm not a sleep doctor, but I have spent years trying to figure out why I wasn't able to sleep better. I've since been fortunate enough to have fixed the exact same problems with hundreds of players and athletes I've worked with over the years. There's really only one secret you need to know about sleep. This secret? It's not about sleep quantity; it's about sleep quality!

Before I get into how to improve your overall sleep quality, it's important to first understand the manner in which you're actually evolved to sleep and how things like blue light from your phone screen can stop you failing asleep from a physiological standpoint.

How we've evolved to sleep

Let's start by going off the grid for a week or two. Let's get back to nature for real. Picture yourself leaving all your possessions behind, your digital watch, laptops, phones, and head out to an uninhabited part of the world where we'll live off the land just as our ancestors did. We'll hunt, fish and sleep under the stars. You can even bring your own food, just no electronic devices.

So, out here in this part of the world, we set up a camp. When the sun eventually goes down, and the temperature drops with it, we build a fire and catch up on what happened during the day. Eventually, after an hour of eating and chatting, the conversation gradually starts to subside and, one by one, we turn over, curl up under our blankets or sleeping bags and drift into sleep.

At some point in the morning, depending the time of year and the part of the world we're in, the sun is going to start approaching the horizon. The birds start singing even before that, and when the sun does start to come out, the temperature begins to rise. Even if it's really cold, it will still rise by a couple of degrees and everything will get brighter. Irrespective of whether we're all wrapped up in our sleeping bags, the natural light gets in and we wake up. The first thing we're likely to want to do is relieve ourselves and empty our bladders, after which we'll start thinking about food and what to have for breakfast. Before long, it'll be time for our morning bowel movement. Nothing rushed or hurried, all in its own time. This is how we're evolved to fall asleep and wake up; but to be honest, I've only experienced this exact scenario when I completed the 250 km Marathon Des Sables in April 2018. This is a self-sufficient six-day event in which you run a marathon each day in the Sahara Desert. With the exception of hunting for food, this was exactly how my routine was for eight days straight (I spent eight nights in the desert in total).

It was the first time I had experienced the complete absence of electronics and artificial light (it was in the middle of the desert after all) and every night, without fail, I fell asleep around 8/8:30 p.m. and woke up every morning with the sun at 5 a.m. Generally, I don't need that many hours of sleep but running a marathon a day in 40-50 degree heat made me more tired than usual, so I generally needed an extra hour or two each night to recover. However, the weirdest thing happened while I was there. Even though I was running a marathon a day for six days straight and had to carry all my food on my back under tumultuous conditions – sand storms, water rations, etc. – because I was falling asleep when the sun went down and waking up when it came up, I actually slept better in the desert than I had at any point in my life! It was an experience that got me extremely interested in understanding more about our natural circadian rhythm. Mentally, I had prepared myself for eight nights of terrible sleep, but the opposite happened. I ended up falling asleep at 8 p.m., sleeping right through the night and waking up directly with the sun at 5 a.m., feeling fully refreshed or at least as refreshed as you could feel after running a marathon in the desert the previous day.

The circadian rhythm

I also spoke about the circadian rhythm in *The Fitness Mindset* and how to avoid the 'night-time second wind' – that surge of energy that comes at night time, keeps your brain awake and stops you from falling asleep. I'll discuss it further in the chapter, as they're linked. But one thing I want to cover first is the circadian rhythm.

One of the first things I do with players who are chronically poor sleepers is ask them, 'Are you aware of the circadian rhythms?' Most have heard of it but aren't sure what it means, and there's a good chance that if you're someone who falls into the bracket of being a poor sleeper, you may not understand it fully either. Thus, hopefully, this helps to explain it in a little more detail.

A circadian rhythm is a 24-hour internal cycle managed by our body clocks. This clock of ours, which functions deep within the brain, regulates our internal systems, such as sleeping and eating patterns, hormone production, mood, digestion, etc., all in a 24-hour process that has evolved to work in sync with the earth's rotation. Your internal body clock is set by external cues, daylight being the main factor. It's vital to understand that this circadian rhythm is hardwired into your DNA and is the by-product of million and millions of years of evolution. Trying to change your circadian rhythm is like asking a fish to get out of the water immediately and learn to fly or asking a lion to convert to veganism. The best direct example you may have experienced as a result of your circadian rhythm is when you travel across different time zones and experience a form of 'jet lag'. When you go from the southern hemisphere to the northern hemisphere for example, your body gets confused between night and day. This is why you're so tired during the day and wired through the night. Your body does reset back to normal, and your internal body clock will self-adjust in the new country once it goes through a few days of the day/light cycles. This phenomenon demonstrates how hardwired this system really is.

The reason that I was able to sleep very early and so well in the Sahara was because once the sun goes down, your body starts to produce a hormone known as melatonin. Melatonin is the hormone that regulates our sleep. It's produced in your pineal gland and responds to light. Once it's been dark long enough, we produce melatonin naturally and we're ready to sleep. According to Nick Littlehales, 'Our body isn't the only regulator of sleep. If we think of circadian rhythms as being our *urge* to sleep, then our homeostatic sleep pressure is our *need* to sleep.' This intuitive 'need' starts building as soon as we wake up and becomes greater the longer we stay awake. That's why you're generally fresher in the morning or mid-morning than in the day, say around lunchtime or in the evening, as you've been awake for longer. However, our circadian rhythm is able to override this at times, and this is the reason that we experience the 'night-time second wind' I spoke about earlier. Any one that's ever worked a night shift or pulled an all-nighter for an exam can attest to this – even though you're exhausted after a full night of work, your body and brain still struggle to fall asleep during the day, as you're fighting your body's circadian urge to be up with the sun. There are a couple of sleep hacks that night workers can use but, truthfully, they can be used by anyone who struggles with sleep in general. Personally, I use all of these nearly every night to ensure I get better sleep quality each night.

Sleep hacks for night workers

1. Black-out blinds: Get blinds that completely block out all natural sunlight in your bedroom. The key is trying to recreate the night darkness in your room – if the sun is shining through your window, you are a going to struggle to fall asleep or stay asleep.

2. Black-out curtains: Normally, these or black-out blinds suffice but, personally, I use both to completely black out my bedroom.

3. Cut the screen time an hour before sleep: This is good advice regardless of what time you go to sleep. I also use 'blue light-blocking glasses' if I want to watch a movie or series before bed. I'll get into blue light later on in the chapter but, for now, cutting back on

'melatonin-stopping blue light' can help you fall asleep more easily after having worked a night shift.

4. <u>Fake a night-time routine:</u> It can be difficult as a night shift worker to have a night-time routine, as you're coming home when everybody else is getting up or still asleep. Routines are very powerful in subconsciously switching off from the day's events (or night, in this case). Try and go to bed the same time every day and keep the routine similar. For example, get home at 7 a.m., eat, have a shower, watch an hour of TV, brush your teeth, go to your blacked out room and sleep from 10 a.m. to 6 p.m. This is just an example, so you can adjust for your lifestyle and preferences.

Is blue light negatively affecting your sleep?

Although there are other factors, light is the most important time-setter for our body clocks, and there are very few things better than the daylight in the morning to help prepare you to wake up and go about your day. In the Sahara, sleeping under the sky, I got my fix as soon as I woke but, in the real world, it's very easy to spend our time indoors – at home, on the train or at our place of work and, especially in Ireland, overcast days are normally supported by artificial lights at home or in the office. My advice is to open your curtains open as soon as you wake up or use a daylight alarm clock that mimics daylight and wakes you by light instead of by alarm – I use one of these religiously in the winter and can say that it is great for anyone that is affected by SAD (seasonal affective disorder), whereby your mood is negatively affected in the winter months from a lack of sunlight.

We are particularly sensitive to a wavelength known as blue light. This is the light that is emitted from electronic devices such as laptops, computers and smartphones. It's not that blue light is bad for you. Daylight from sun is full of blue light and, during the day, blue light helps keep you alert and awake. It naturally sets your body clock, suppresses melatonin production and keeps you focused throughout the day. However, can you see how all those positive traits from during the day can quickly become negative if you're planning to sleep in the next few hours? There's a great term used by sleep expert Chris Idzikowski called 'junk sleep' – this is when, even though you may be getting the traditional eight hours of sleep, the gadgets inhibit the production of melatonin and push our body clocks further – which is another possible reason that you can wake up feeling groggy and tired. This is why I felt so exhausted for years regardless of what supplements or night-time routines I used, and if you're consistently waking up tired, it's probably due to the same thing. It's worth noting that the yellows, ambers and reds that radiate from a fire don't affect melatonin. The reason for this is that the fires and candle light don't negatively affect your sleep, but the blue light from screens does.

How to supplement-hack your sleep

For some, minimising blue light and caffeine or stimulants closer to bedtime is enough to get a great night's sleep. However, if you find yourself really needing a supercharge, there are some supplements that will work wonders for you by either helping you fall asleep or keeping you in a deeper sleep.

Always check your supplements to verify their compatibility with medications that you may be taking, as some vitamins and minerals have been known to reduce the effect of some medications such as birth control pills. There are a number of great herbs and supplements that can help you get a great night's sleep.

Here are some that I've found support me the best and that don't leave me feeling groggy in the morning. Getting a good night's sleep is great; but if you wake up feeling foggy, it defeats the entire purpose.

Zinc: This is an important supplement for male and female fertility and thereby aids libido as well, as zinc deficiency can lead to lower testosterone levels. Both men and women need balanced testosterone levels for optimal hormonal support. Zinc can support testosterone production by putting you into a deeper sleep, which also dramatically improves recovery for athletes, as zinc is one of the first minerals to get depleted in the bodies of gym-goers and athletes.

Dosage: It is normally best taken at a dosage of 25 mg per day with magnesium (see below) and vitamin B6 (ZMA) about 30 minutes before bed on an empty stomach.

Magnesium: Nowadays, nearly everyone is deficient in magnesium. Refined/processed foods are stripped off their mineral, vitamin and fibre content. These are anti-nutrient foods because they actually steal magnesium in order to get metabolised. When consumed, if not supplemented with magnesium, we become increasingly deficient.

Are you tense and tight or crave chocolate? Anything that makes you tense or tight could be potentially due to a magnesium deficiency, which is one reason why you may crave chocolate at night-time or when stressed. Chocolate has one of the highest magnesium content of all food sources. The case of consuming chocolate is a catch-22 though. Even though it has magnesium, chocolate also has sugar. Every molecule of sugar you consume pulls over 50 times the amount of magnesium out of the body. This is only the case with milk chocolate, however. 85% or more dark chocolate retains its high magnesium content and is a great snack food to include in nearly any dietary plan.

Dosage Try taking 600-800 mg a day 30 minutes before bed. However, be careful, as too much too soon can upset your stomach. When you find the correct dosage, due to its mild effect on your central nervous system, you will find that you are much more relaxed when going to bed.

GABA: An inhibitory neurotransmitter, your brain uses GABA to shut itself down. It can dramatically calm you down when taken on an empty stomach. I normally take it 60 minutes after my meal. GABA is great at bed time, but can also be used during the day if you're highly stressed or dealing with anxiety.

Dosage: Start with 500 mg before bed. This dosage can go as high as 2,500 mg (steadily incrementing the dose).

EPILOGUE

Writing this book has been one of the most enjoyable professional experiences of my life. Although my first book, *The Fitness Mindset*, spent eight straight weeks on the bestseller list and was a passion project of mine, *Leaner, Stronger, Faster* was a real labour of love. For me, this was the book I always wanted while I was still playing and the book I would have given anything to read when I was in my early twenties. If your goal is to become the very best player you can possibly be, but also achieve a leaner (or bigger) body that makes you feel more confident when stepping onto the pitch or even walking into any room, bar or club, then that's what I hope this book does for you. I wanted to create a piece of work that you could refer to over and over again, which would help you with nutrition, training, supplements and sleep. I hope it serves as your reference going forward. Of course, it's impossible for me to make it 100% applicable to every single individual, as one person's starting point, sport, gender and goals are going to be extremely different from the next. However, I've gone with rules that are applicable to the majority and best practices for nearly all cases, so I hope you enjoyed reading. If the book helped you, please pass it on or recommend it to your friends, family or teammates. Thank you for reading.

Brian

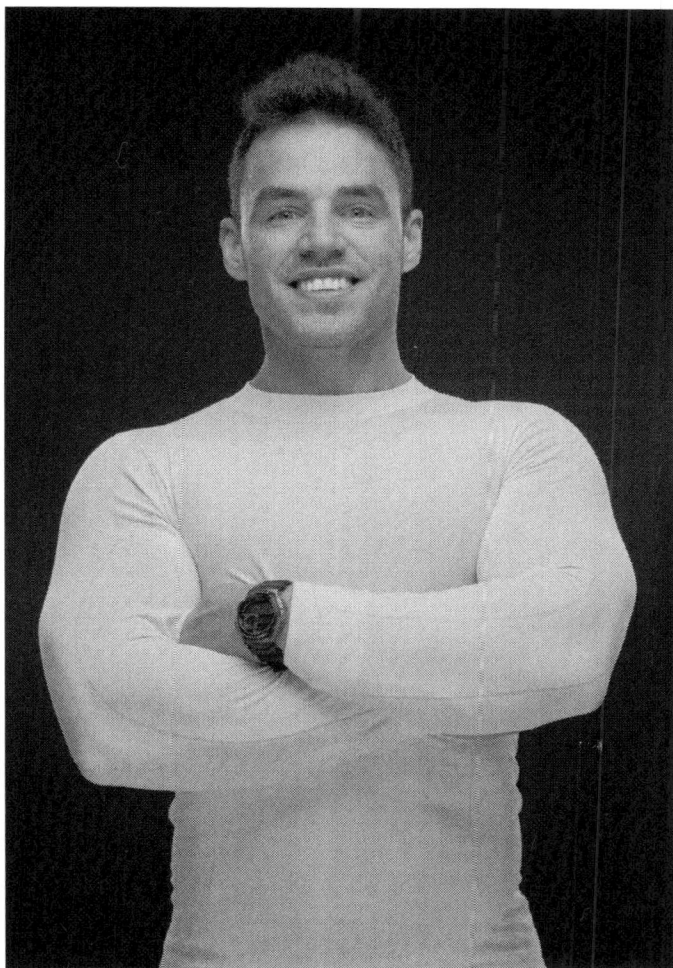

ABOUT THE AUTHOR

Brian Keane is a strength/conditioning coach and sports nutritionist. He has worked with everyone from underage athletes to top inter-county players. Having played GAA for most of his life, he now competes in ultra-endurance events all around the world.

To work with Brian in one of his GAA programs or to follow his content, check out his website www.briankeanefitness.com or search for his social media channels and podcasts through your favourite search engine.